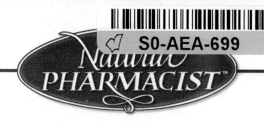

**Natural PHARMACIST™**

## Inside—Find the Answers to These Questions and More

☑ How can I tell if I'm at risk for a heart attack? (See page 10.)

☑ Is it true that I might have heart disease and no symptoms? (See page xi.)

☑ If I've already had a heart attack, are there ways I can prevent another one? (See page xi.)

☑ Can soy protein help reduce my cholesterol? (See page 76.)

☑ Can certain minerals help reduce high blood pressure? (See page 135.)

☑ Can niacin supplements reduce my risk of heart attack? (See page 58.)

☑ Can vitamin E prevent heart disease? (See page 89.)

☑ Can garlic really lower cholesterol levels and high blood pressure? (See page 68.)

☑ Can B vitamins help prevent heart disease? (See page 106.)

☑ How can I stop heart disease before it starts? (See page 12.)

# THE NATURAL PHARMACIST Library

Arthritis

Diabetes

Echinacea and Immunity

Feverfew and Migraines

Garlic and Cholesterol

Ginkgo and Memory

Heart Disease Prevention

Herbs

Illnesses and Their Natural Remedies

Kava and Anxiety

Menopause

PMS

Reducing Cancer Risk

Saw Palmetto and the Prostate

St. John's Wort and Depression

Vitamins and Supplements

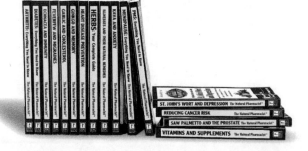

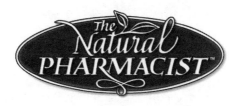

**Everything You Need to Know About**

# Heart Disease Prevention

## Richard Harkness, Pharm., FASCP

*Series Editors*

Steven Bratman, M.D.

David Kroll, Ph.D.

A DIVISION OF PRIMA PUBLISHING

Visit us online at www.thenaturalpharmacist.com

### Warning—Disclaimer

**This book is not intended to provide medical advice and is sold with the understanding that the publisher and the author are not liable for the misconception or misuse of information provided. The author and Prima Publishing shall have neither liability nor responsibility to any person or entity with respect to any loss, damage, or injury caused or alleged to be caused directly or indirectly by the information contained in this book or the use of any products mentioned. Readers should not use any of the products discussed in this book without the advice of a medical professional.**

**The Food and Drug Administration has not approved the use of any of the natural treatments discussed in this book. This book and the information contained herein, has not been approved by the Food and Drug Administration.**

Pseudonyms are used throughout to protect the privacy of individuals involved.

PRIMA HEALTH and colophon are trademarks of Prima Communications, Inc.

THE NATURAL PHARMACIST™ is a trademark of Prima Communications, Inc.

All products mentioned in this book are trademarks of their respective companies.

**Library of Congress Cataloging-in-Publication Data**

Harkness, Richard.
    Heart disease prevention / Richard Harkness.
        p.    cm.–(The natural pharmacist)
    Includes bibliographical references and index.
    ISBN 0-7615-1731-6
    1. Heart—Diseases—Diet therapy—Popular works.    2. Heart—Diseases—Prevention—Nutritional aspects—Popular works.
    I. Title.    II. Series.
RC684.D5H37    1998
616.1'205—dc21                                                                98-53498
                                                                                      CIP

00 01 02 03 04  HH 10 9 8 7 6 5 4 3
Printed in the United States of America

**Visit us online at www.thenaturalpharmacist.com**

# Contents

*What Makes This Book Different?*   *vii*
*Introduction*   *xi*

1. About Heart Disease   1

2. The ABCs of Cholesterol and Triglycerides   15

3. Guidelines for Managing Your Cholesterol   20

4. Conventional Therapies for High Cholesterol   25

5. Niacin and High Cholesterol   55

6. Garlic and High Cholesterol   66

7. Other Natural Therapies for High Cholesterol   75

8. Vitamin E and Other Antioxidants   87

9. Homocysteine and Heart Disease   103

10. Using B Vitamins to Control
    High Homocysteine   106

11. High Blood Pressure and Heart Disease   115

12. Conventional Therapies for
    High Blood Pressure   121

13. Nutrients and Herbs That Lower
    High Blood Pressure   134

14. Putting It All Together   146

    *Notes*   154
    *Index*   179
    *About the Author and Series Editors*   193

# What Makes This Book Different?

The interest in natural medicine has never been greater. According to the National Association of Chain Drug Stores, 65 million Americans are using natural supplements, and the number is growing! Yet, it is hard for the consumer to find trustworthy sources for balanced information about this emerging field. Why? Frankly, natural medicine has had a checkered history. From snake oil potions sold at the turn of the century to those books, magazines, and product catalogs that hype miracle cures today, this is a field where exaggerated claims have been the norm. Proponents of natural medicine have tended to abuse science, treating it more as a marketing tool than a means of discovering the truth.

But there is truth to be found. Studies of vitamins, minerals, and other food supplements have been with us since these nutritional substances were first discovered, and the level and quality of this science has grown dramatically in the last 20 years. Herbal medicine has been neglected in the United States, but in Europe, this, the oldest of all healing arts, has been the subject of tremendous and ongoing scientific interest.

At present, for a number of herbs and supplements, it is possible to give reasonably scientific answers to the questions: How well does this work? How safe is it? What types of conditions is it best used for?

THE NATURAL PHARMACIST series is designed to cut through the hype and tell you what we know and what we don't know about popular natural treatments. These books are more conservative than any others available, more honest about the weaknesses of natural approaches, more fair in their comparisons of natural and conventional treatments. You won't find any miracle cures here, but you will discover useful options that can help you become healthier.

## Why Choose Natural Treatments?

Although the science behind natural medicine continues to grow, this is still a much less scientifically validated field than conventional medicine. You might ask, "Why should I resort to an herb that is only partly proven, when I could take a drug with solid science behind it?" There are at least three good reasons to consider natural alternatives.

First, some herbs and supplements offer benefits that are not matched by any conventional drug. Vitamin E is a good example. It appears to help prevent prostate cancer, a benefit that no standard medication can claim. Also, vitamin E almost certainly helps prevent heart disease. While there are standard drugs that also prevent heart disease, vitamin E works differently and may be able to complement many of the other approaches.

Another example is the herb milk thistle. Studies strongly suggest that this herb can protect the liver from injury. There is no pill or tablet your doctor can prescribe to do the same.

Even if the science behind some of these treatments is less than perfect, when the risks are low and the possible benefit high, a natural treatment may be worth trying. It is a little-known fact that for many conventional treatments the science is less than perfect as well, and physicians must balance uncertain benefits against incompletely understood risks.

A second reason to consider natural therapies is that some may offer benefits comparable to those of drugs with fewer side effects. The herb St. John's wort is a good example. Reasonably strong scientific evidence suggests that this herb is an effective treatment for mild to moderate depression, while producing fewer side effects on average than conventional medications. Saw palmetto for benign enlargement of the prostate, ginkgo for relieving symptoms and perhaps slowing the progression of Alzheimer's disease, and glucosamine for osteoarthritis are other examples. This is not to say that herbs and supplements are completely harmless—they're not—but for most the level of risk is quite low.

Finally, there is a philosophical point to consider. For many people, it "feels" better to use a treatment that comes from nature instead of from a laboratory. Just as you might rather wear all-cotton clothing than polyester, or look at a mountain landscape rather than the skyscrapers of a downtown city, natural treatments may simply feel more compatible with your view of life. We can quibble endlessly about just what "natural" means and whether a certain treatment is "actually" natural or not, but such arguments are beside the point. The difference is in the feeling, and feelings matter. In fact, having a good feeling about taking an herb may lead you to use it more consistently than you would a prescription drug.

Of course, at times synthetic drugs may be necessary and even lifesaving. But on many other occasions it may be quite reasonable to turn to an herb or supplement instead of a drug.

To make good decisions you need good information. Unfortunately, while hundreds of books on alternative medicine are published every year, many are highly misleading.

The phrase "studies prove" is often used when the studies in question are so small or so badly conducted that they prove nothing at all. You may even find that the "data" from other books comes from studies with petri dishes and not real people!

You can't even assume that books written by well-known authors are scientifically sound. Many of these authors rely on secondary writers, leading to a game of "telephone," where misconceptions are passed around from book to book. And there's a strong tendency to exaggerate the power of natural remedies, whitewashing them with selective reporting.

THE NATURAL PHARMACIST series gives you the balanced information you need to make informed decisions about your health needs. Setting a new, high standard of accuracy and objectivity, these books take a realistic look at the herbs and supplements you read about in the news. You will encounter both favorable and unfavorable studies in these pages and will learn about both the benefits and the risks of natural treatments.

THE NATURAL PHARMACIST series is the source you can trust.

Steven Bratman, M.D.
David Kroll, Ph.D.

# Introduction

**Y**our heart is a unique organ. It pumps life to all other organs in your body, including itself. Perhaps that's one reason it's been endowed with qualities transcending its mechanical function—historically and poetically, the heart has been regarded as the seat of our feelings and emotions.

*The Natural Pharmacist Guide to Heart Disease Prevention* shows you how to protect this vital little pump from its number one enemy: heart disease. Doing that will add many healthy and productive years to your life.

If you have already suffered and survived the dire consequences of heart disease, such as heart attack or stroke, the information in this book will help you avoid another such event. If you have active heart disease with angina pain or other symptoms, you'll find out how to lower your risk of further progression and perhaps even coax its retreat.

Heart disease (coronary artery disease) stands alone as the number one disease killer in the United States and most other industrialized countries. Treacherously, it progresses without symptoms for decades, attacking the arteries that carry blood to the heart itself. Deposits called plaque build up inside these arteries, narrowing them so that less blood is able to flow through. For some, the first sign of heart disease is the severe chest pain called angina; but for others, it's the jolt of a sudden, possibly fatal, heart attack or stroke.

Primary prevention means stopping heart disease before it starts or progresses to clinical disease. Secondary prevention means halting its progression in people who already have it. The line between the primary and secondary prevention is blurred for several reasons. First, heart disease may begin in childhood, progressing silently for decades before clogging arteries enough to show itself. Also, the methods used in secondary prevention—controlling primary risk factors such as high cholesterol levels and high blood pressure—also work as primary preventives. Simply put, prevention appears to work at whatever stage you start.

We'll cover both conventional and alternative methods to control your risk factors. Information on conventional methods—eating better, quitting smoking, exercising, losing weight, and drug therapy—is widely available from many sources. In contrast, reliable, scientific information on using nature's finely tuned botanical orchestra of nutrients and herbs is hard to come by, and that will be our emphasis.

Here, for the first time, the cutting-edge research evidence on the use of natural supplements to prevent heart disease has been gathered in one place, then analyzed and interpreted so it's easy to understand. *The Natural Pharmacist Guide to Heart Disease Prevention* is your unique guide through the research thicket.

We'll focus our preventive crosshairs on three primary risk factors: high cholesterol levels, high blood pressure, and high homocysteine levels. Numerous studies suggest these risk factors can, in many cases, be managed with selected natural agents such as vitamins, minerals, amino acids, and herbs. We'll also look at the role of antioxidants such as vitamin E in preventing heart disease. This book sorts the wheat from the chaff, telling you what's mostly hype and what really works.

The supplements in our spotlight include niacin, garlic, vitamins E and C, vitamins $B_6$, $B_{12}$, and folic acid, magnesium and other minerals, soy protein, sitostanol, red yeast rice, tocotrienols, fish oil, flaxseed oil, coenzyme $Q_{10}$, carnitine, hawthorn, ginkgo biloba, bilberry, selenium, green tea, khella, pantethine, gugulipid, and ginseng. Some of the research results excite even stoic researchers, and hints at intriguing possibilities for eventual natural prevention of this most widespread and deadly disease.

A new study published in the *Lancet* found that fully half of American men and one-third of women under age 40 will develop heart disease over their lifetimes.[1] In the past it was thought that those who reached age 70 without heart disease were probably not going to develop it. This study suggests otherwise, that the risk remains significantly high even for individuals who reach 70 still free of the disease.

These findings bring home two important points:

- Treating so many people with medications is simply not an acceptable way to manage the modern epidemic of heart disease.
- Preventing heart disease is the key, and the sooner you start, the better.

In this book you will find the best currently available information on effective and practical ways to protect yourself from heart disease using natural methods. Take the information in this book to heart, and you and your family will be on the wellness road to longer, healthier lives.

# About Heart Disease

**Y**our cardiovascular system consists of an intricate network of blood vessels and the seemingly tireless organ called the heart. This system is a closed loop, with the heart as its hub. Blood vessels called arteries carry blood from the heart to the body, while blood vessels called veins carry blood back to the heart.

The heart first pumps blood through your lungs, where it releases carbon dioxide and replenishes itself with fresh oxygen from the air we breathe. From the lungs, the blood flows to the rest of your body, depositing oxygen and nutrients to organs and tissues. The depleted blood then returns to your heart, and the life-preserving cycle repeats itself. It's easy to see how a kink in this system can cause serious problems.

Unless otherwise noted, when we talk about heart disease, we're referring to coronary artery disease or CAD, which involves the arteries that supply blood to the heart itself. In CAD, these arteries have become so narrow they can no longer supply enough blood to meet your heart's demand for the oxygen it needs to function properly. The narrowing is usually the result of an underlying disease process called atherosclerosis. For this reason, it is also called atherosclerotic heart disease.

The common term for atherosclerosis is hardening of the arteries. *Atherosclerosis* comes from the Greek words *athero* (gruel or paste) and *sklerosis* (hardness).

The condition is characterized by the buildup of plaque (deposits containing fat and other substances) within the interior wall of an artery. Over time, this causes the artery wall to swell, partially blocking the space through which blood flows.

When your heart fails to get enough oxygen, it signals its plight with the severe pain called *angina*. When this occurs without pain, it's called *silent ischemia* (ischemia is an oxygen deficiency). A complete blockage or severe restriction of the arteries feeding the heart causes a heart attack. As described below, this is usually due to a combination of atherosclerosis and a blood clot. *Congestive heart failure* often follows damage from a heart attack, which leaves the heart too weak to adequately pump blood to the rest of the body. An *arrhythmia* (irregular heart rhythm) may occur when oxygen deprivation—again, from either ischemia or a heart attack—damages heart cells that carry heart-regulating electrical impulses. A critical arrhythmia can result in sudden death.

Atherosclerosis causes more than heart disease; it is also the disease process underlying cerebrovascular disease (CVD) and peripheral arterial disease (PAD). All these disorders share a common link: atherosclerosis in the arteries that feed tissues of the body. In the case of coronary artery disease, the blood-deprived part is the heart itself. In cerebrovascular disease, it's the brain. In peripheral arterial disease, it's the body's extremities (causing, for example, intermittent claudication—severe pain in calf muscles during walking or exercising). By preventing coronary artery disease, you also prevent stroke and other atherosclerosis-related conditions.

Next we'll take a look deep into arteries to see how atherosclerotic heart disease develops. This will help us better understand the preventive methods we'll be discussing later.

## What Causes Heart Disease?

As we've seen, coronary artery disease results from the buildup of plaque inside the interior walls of the arteries supplying blood and nutrients to the heart itself. The plaque buildup (atherosclerosis) begins in childhood and progresses silently behind the scenes, declaring itself only after it has advanced enough to produce symptoms—usually during middle age or later. Several studies have shown that signs of atherosclerosis can be found in children as early as 1 year old. By age 10, almost all children show some indication of fatty streaks, a telltale sign of early atherosclerosis.[1] We know this disease process is accelerated by high cholesterol, high blood pressure, diabetes, smoking, physical inactivity, and possibly by high homocysteine levels.

**The plaque buildup (atherosclerosis) begins in childhood and progresses silently behind the scenes, declaring itself only after it has advanced enough to produce symptoms—usually during middle age or later.**

Bacterial infections, such as *H. pylori* and *Chlamydia*, may also contribute to the development of heart disease.

Atherosclerotic lesions in some people have been found to harbor a form of *Chlamydia* that causes pneumonia, and researchers have determined that the infection preceded the atherosclerotic damage.[2] Other research has hinted that periodontitis—a dental inflammation—may be associated with heart disease, but this is not firmly established.[3]

Though much remains unclear, the basic process of atherosclerosis has come into sharper focus. The first step is injury to the endothelium, the delicate layer of cells lining the inner walls of arteries. Various factors may contribute to this injury. The direct mechanical stress of high blood pressure can, over time, damage the artery wall. Cholesterol, homocysteine, elevated blood sugar, nicotine (from smoking), and free radicals also appear to play a role. Areas of high turbulence, such as where arteries branch off, are especially prone to injury. This damaged, inflamed area is the rallying point for a cascade of events leading to plaque formation.

**We know this disease process is accelerated by high cholesterol, high blood pressure, diabetes, smoking, physical inactivity, and possibly by high homocysteine levels.**

Simply put, microscopic debris begins to accumulate inside the tissue of the inner artery wall. Over time, this debris causes the wall to bulge outward and creates an ever larger speed bump that obstructs blood flow. During this process, LDL cholesterol (the bad kind) becomes oxidized and contributes to further injury and plaque growth. Fatty streaks, mentioned earlier, represent the early stages of these changes, and are the first identifiable stage in plaque formation.

Smaller lesions "connect" to form what is called *complicated plaque.* Complicated plaque continues to grow in both size and thickness until the artery becomes partially or completely blocked or until the artery wall becomes so weak that it ruptures. Partial blockage tends to cause reversible symptoms such as angina, intermittent claudication, and TIAs or transient ischemic attacks (often referred to as "mini-strokes"). Plaque may start to break away from the thin vessel wall, resulting in small areas of bleeding. The clotting system responds by forming thrombi (blood clots) at the bleeding sites. Clots may also form simply because the surface of the plaque is ragged. At this stage, the danger is much more than local. Either a piece of plaque or a blood clot can splinter off and form a logjam in an artery downstream, resulting in a full-blown heart attack or stroke.

## The Consequences: Heart Attack and Stroke

We've already mentioned the serious conditions resulting from atherosclerosis. Let's look at them in more detail.

### Angina

Angina refers to severe chest pain caused by restricted blood flow to your heart, usually due to arteries narrowed by heart disease. A less common cause is spasm of coronary arteries. Angina may be triggered by activity, extreme cold, stress, or even a large meal. The pain usually goes away at rest, because a resting heart requires less oxygen.

Angina can take many forms. The pain is usually perceived as a dull, heavy pressure in the center of your chest and may radiate to the neck, jaw, left shoulder, or arm. You may also have shortness of breath, palpitations, weakness, or faintness.

If your arteries are clogged enough to cause angina pain, you are at severe risk for a heart attack. In this sense, angina can be viewed as a kind of warning. As we'll see in later chapters, it may be possible for you to reverse your heart disease, preventing a future heart attack and even eliminating angina.

Along with medications, the best treatment for angina is to reduce as many cardiac risk factors as you can: get control of your cholesterol, blood pressure, and homocysteine levels, improve your diet, increase your physical activity, and quit smoking. There are many natural treatments that can help you with some of these important steps.

## Silent Ischemia

If you have silent ischemia (ischemia is an oxygen deficiency), you won't get any warning pain or other symptoms. People with diabetes are particularly susceptible to this form of ischemia. This condition can be a greater threat than angina, since you don't know to seek help. Fortunately, like angina, silent ischemia produces abnormalities that can be recognized on an electrocardiogram. For this reason, you should get regular electrocardiograms if you have diabetes or other risk factors for heart disease.

## Heart Attack

The gravest consequence of heart disease is a heart attack (myocardial infarction). A heart attack occurs when blood flow through a coronary artery is completely blocked or severely restricted, usually by a blood clot. The areas of the heart deprived of blood die and cause the heart to lose some of its function.

Of the 1.5 million people who suffer a heart attack yearly in the United States, about 300,000 die before getting appropriate medical care.[4] Another 200,000 die within the first month, most within 24 hours of admission. Unfortunately, a

## Warning Signs of Heart Attack

Immediately call for emergency help if you or someone nearby experiences any of the following symptoms:[5]

- An uncomfortable pressure, fullness, squeezing, or pain in the center of the chest that lasts longer than 15 minutes.
- Severe chest pain.
- Pain spreading to the shoulders, neck, or arms.
- Lightheadedness and palpitations.
- Fainting.
- Sweating or nausea associated with chest discomfort.
- Difficulty breathing.

The sooner a heart attack receives medical attention, the greater your chances for survival and for minimizing damage to your heart.

first heart attack may occur with no warning and is often fatal. The risk increases dramatically with age. Women are more likely than men to die from heart attacks, and African Americans are more likely to die than Caucasians. The Framingham Heart Study recorded 5% of heart attacks in individuals under age 40, and 45% in those under 65. Almost 80% of deaths occurred in those 65 and older.

Heart attacks require conventional treatment. The best use of natural medicine is to help prevent them.

## Congestive Heart Failure

Congestive heart failure (CHF) is often simply called heart failure. The leading causes of heart failure are injury to the heart from heart attacks and high blood pressure.

Damage from a heart attack significantly increases your risk of heart failure.[6] The Framingham study indicated that heart failure developed in 23% of men and 35% of women who survived a heart attack. That rate is four to eight times higher than the incidence of heart failure in people who have not experienced a heart attack. A heart attack kills heart muscle cells, replacing them with scar tissue. The more cells lost, the weaker and less able the heart is to pump blood to the far reaches of the body.

High blood pressure (discussed in chapter 11) requires your heart muscle to enlarge so it can pump harder, and over time this weakens it. In this case, lowering your blood pressure may halt the progression of heart failure.

Because a weakened heart cannot pump out all the blood it receives, blood backs up and pools in your veins. Pooling in the lungs results in shortness of breath. Pooling in the abdomen and legs produces swelling (edema). Heart failure can make you too weak and fatigued to engage in your usual activities. It's also the leading reason for hospitalization of the elderly.

## Stroke

Stroke is another serious consequence of atherosclerosis. In fact, stroke causes more long-term disability than any other disease.[7] As with a heart attack, a stroke occurs when the blood supply is cut off—in this case, to your brain. That's why it's called a "brain attack." Although stroke is not the primary subject of this book, it is closely linked to heart attacks.

The two primary types of stroke are ischemic stroke and hemorrhagic stroke. Ischemic stroke, the most common type, results when an artery supplying blood to your brain is blocked, usually by a piece of plaque that has broken off from its primary site. A hemorrhagic stroke occurs when an artery in your brain bursts and floods the surrounding

## Warning Signs of Stroke

Call for emergency help immediately if you or someone nearby experiences any of the following symptoms:[8]

- Sudden weakness or numbness of the face, arm, or leg on one side of the body.
- Sudden dimness or loss of vision, particularly in one eye.
- Loss of speech, or trouble talking or understanding speech.
- Sudden severe headaches with no apparent cause.
- Unexplained dizziness, unsteadiness, or sudden falls, especially along with any of the previous symptoms.

The sooner a stroke receives medical attention, the greater your chances for survival and for minimizing damage to your brain.

tissue with blood. Ischemic strokes are often preceded by "mini-strokes," or TIAs, which can be due to small wandering clots called emboli or simply to impaired circulation. In the elderly, TIAs may account for many treatable and preventable cases of senile dementia, which might otherwise be diagnosed as Alzheimer's disease.

If the disruption of blood flow lasts too long, brain tissue begins to die. Whatever function the damaged area of the brain enabled will be impaired—for example, speech, vision, or movement.

In the United States, half a million people suffer a stroke yearly and almost 150,000 die. About 71% of stroke victims continue to have impaired vocational ability 7 years later, according to the AHA. The risk of stroke doubles every 10 years after age 55, and men have a 19% higher risk than women. Due to high rates of high blood pressure in African Americans, blacks are twice as likely as whites to suffer a stroke, often at a younger age and with more severity. The good news is that the overall death rate from stroke has plunged since 1950, perhaps due to better medical treatment and increased public awareness of the need to seek immediate help.

# Are You at Risk for Heart Disease?

The more overall risk factors you have, the greater the chance you will develop heart disease. According to the AHA, these are the primary or major risk factors for coronary artery disease:

- Age
- Male sex
- Heredity (including race)
- Smoking
- High blood cholesterol levels
- High blood pressure
- Physical inactivity
- Obesity and overweight
- Diabetes mellitus
- Stress (may be a contributing factor)

You're stuck with the built-in risk factors—age, gender, and heredity—these first three can't be changed. But you can modify or control the other primary risk factors. Let's look at the risk factors more closely, courtesy of AHA.

## Increasing Age

About four out of five people who die of coronary artery disease are age 65 or older. At older ages, women who have heart attacks are twice as likely as men are to die from them within a few weeks.

## Male Sex

Men have a greater risk of heart attack than women, and they have attacks earlier in life. Even after menopause, when women's death rate from heart disease increases, it's not as great as men's.

## Heredity (Including Race)

Children of parents with heart disease are more likely to develop it themselves. African Americans have more severe hypertension than whites. Consequently, their risk of heart disease is greater.

## Cigarette and Tobacco Smoking

A smoker's risk of heart attack is more than twice that of non-smokers. Cigarette smoking is the biggest risk factor for sudden cardiac death: Smokers have two to four times the risk of nonsmokers. Smokers who have a heart attack are more likely to die and die suddenly (within an hour) than are nonsmokers. Available evidence also indicates that chronic exposure to environmental tobacco smoke (secondhand smoke, passive smoking) may increase the risk of heart disease.

## High Blood Cholesterol Levels

The risk of coronary artery disease rises as blood cholesterol levels increase. When other risk factors (such as high blood pressure and cigarette smoke) are present, this risk increases even more. A person's cholesterol level is also affected by age, sex, heredity, and diet. As we shall see, several natural treatments can lower cholesterol levels, at least one of which has very strong evidence for its effectiveness.

## High Blood Pressure

High blood pressure increases the heart's workload, causing the heart to enlarge and weaken over time. It also increases the risk of stroke, heart attack, kidney failure, and congestive heart failure. When high blood pressure exists with obesity, smoking, high blood cholesterol levels, or diabetes, the risk of heart attack or stroke increases several times. Weaker evidence suggests that some natural treatments may be able to lower blood pressure.

### Physical Inactivity

Lack of physical activity is a risk factor for coronary artery disease. Regular, moderate-to-vigorous exercise plays a significant role in preventing heart and blood vessel disease. Even modest levels of low-intensity physical activity are beneficial if done regularly and long term. Exercise can help control blood cholesterol, diabetes, and obesity, and can help lower blood pressure in some people.

### Obesity and Excess Weight

People who have excess body fat are more likely to develop heart disease and stroke even if they have no other risk factors. Obesity is unhealthy because excess weight increases the strain on the heart. It's directly linked with coronary artery disease because it influences blood pressure, blood cholesterol, and triglyceride levels, and makes diabetes more likely to develop. Losing as little as 10 to 20 pounds will help lower your heart disease risk.

### Diabetes Mellitus

Diabetes seriously increases the risk of developing cardiovascular disease. Even when glucose levels are under control, diabetes significantly increases the risk of heart disease and stroke. More than 80% of people with diabetes die of some form of heart or blood vessel disease. If you have diabetes, it is critically important for you to monitor and control any other risk factors you can.

## What You Can Do

Even if you have all of the risk factors on the list, it is never too late to reduce them. There's not much you can do about your age, gender, and heredity, of course, but the others can be changed. In the rest of this book, we'll look at each of the changeable risk factors and show you what you can do about them to significantly reduce your risk of heart disease and its most serious consequences, including heart attack and stroke.

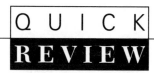

QUICK REVIEW

- Heart disease kills more people in the United States than any other disease.
- Heart disease develops slowly.

    Plaque builds up inside arteries that carry blood to the heart itself.

    Atherosclerosis, the underlying disease process that causes plaque buildup, generally starts during childhood.

    Over time, blood flow becomes impeded, starving your heart of the oxygen and nutrients it needs to do its life-preserving work.

- Angina (heart pain) is a symptom, but the first sign could also be a sudden heart attack.
- Stroke is another serious consequence of atherosclerosis.
- Heart disease is associated with a number of risk factors.

    The controllable causes of heart disease—the major risk factors—are high cholesterol levels, high blood pressure, high homocysteine levels, smoking, physical inactivity, being overweight, and diabetes. Stress may play a contributing role.

    The uncontrollable risk factors of heart disease are age, male sex, heredity, and race.

■ What you'll find in this book:

Conventional methods of prevention.

Cutting-edge research evidence on the use of natural supplements to prevent heart disease.

Easy-to-understand interpretation of the evidence.

Practical information you can start using immediately to protect your heart.

# The ABCs of Cholesterol and Triglycerides

**A**s we saw in chapter 1, atherosclerotic plaques are not merely clumps of fat or cholesterol stuck inside arteries. Cholesterol does, however, play a major role in plaque development. In fact, high levels of cholesterol are a major cause of atherosclerotic heart disease. Another form of fat, triglycerides, also plays a role.

According to the American Heart Association (AHA), as many as 97 million Americans have elevated blood cholesterol levels. Almost 38 million adults exceed levels defined as high risk.

Cholesterol is not inherently bad. Indeed, it's vital for good health. Without it, your body could not make sex hormones, cell membranes, or vitamin D. Cholesterol is also used in the production of bile acids, which are essential to the digestion of fatty foods. The problem is when your cholesterol levels run out of control.

# What Is Cholesterol?

Cholesterol is a waxy, fatty substance called a *lipid.* Your liver manufactures it, as do the livers of all animals. That's why cholesterol is found in eggs, meat, fish, and milk. Since plants don't have livers, you won't find cholesterol in fruits, vegetables, or grains. Consuming a lot of cholesterol in your daily diet can raise your cholesterol levels, but this is not the only factor or even the most important one. For reasons that are not entirely clear, if you eat a lot of animal fat—which is saturated fat—your body raises its own cholesterol levels, and this is generally a more powerful influence.

**Cholesterol is not inherently bad. Indeed, it's vital for good health.**

## LDL and HDL Cholesterol: The Bad and the Good

Just as oil does not mix with water, neither does cholesterol mix with blood, which is mostly water. Since blood shuns plain cholesterol, your liver packages it so it can be ferried through the bloodstream. The packages, called *lipoproteins,* come in various types. The two that are most important appear to be low-density lipoprotein (LDL) and high-density lipoprotein (HDL).

LDL cholesterol is "bad" because it directly contributes to plaque development. In contrast, HDL cholesterol is "good" because higher levels make you less likely to get heart disease. We don't know exactly how HDL cholesterol works, but it appears to help remove cholesterol from your body. It's been suggested that HDL cholesterol may also pick up cholesterol from plaque lesions and thus help stall or reverse them.

## Triglycerides

Another form of fat in the blood is called triglycerides. Although triglycerides play a less important role in the development of heart disease than cholesterol, increased levels of triglycerides apparently do increase the risk of heart disease.[1] The risk grows with increasing triglyceride levels.

## Dyslipidemias: Abnormal Cholesterol Levels

Since cholesterol is a lipid, abnormal levels of the various types of cholesterol are referred to as *dyslipidemias.* Common dyslipidemias include high total cholesterol, high triglycerides, high LDL cholesterol, and low HDL cholesterol. LDL cholesterol is the primary target of lipid-lowering treatment.

# High Cholesterol and You

The evidence that high cholesterol raises the risk of heart disease is convincing. One of the bedrock studies on heart disease is the Framingham Heart Study. It began in 1948 and followed 5,209 people living in Framingham, Massachusetts. The study established a firm connection between cholesterol levels and heart disease in both men and women.[2] It found that, as your total cholesterol levels rise above 200, so does your risk of heart disease. A total cholesterol level of 250 doubles your risk compared to a level of 200. A total cholesterol level of 300 boosts your risk fourfold.

Similarly, the Multiple Risk Factor Intervention Trial (MRFIT) found that your risk of death from heart disease is related to your total cholesterol levels in a continuous, graded fashion.[3] Finally, people with the genetic disorder called *familial hypercholesterolemia* (abnormally high cholesterol levels) tend to develop premature atherosclerosis.

**The evidence that high cholesterol raises the risk of heart disease is convincing. A total cholesterol level of 250 doubles your risk compared to a level of 200. A total cholesterol level of 300 boosts your risk fourfold.**

Added up, the evidence is compelling for a cause-and-effect relationship between high cholesterol and heart disease. Levels of LDL cholesterol seem to be most closely associated with heart disease risk. The earlier you start controlling your cholesterol levels, the better.

If you already have heart disease with symptoms such as angina, or have survived a heart attack, you may not need much convincing to get your cholesterol levels in check. It's especially critical that you do this, because you have a five to seven times greater risk of heart attack than someone without heart disease.[4]

You're likely to be a harder sell on corralling your cholesterol if you have no symptoms of heart disease at all. Here's a sobering fact that may act as a jumpstart: One-fifth of coronary deaths occur in people with no history of heart disease, and these deaths can't be predicted by risk factors.[5]

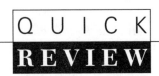

QUICK
REVIEW

- Cholesterol is a key factor in heart disease, but it is also vital to good health.

The problem occurs when cholesterol levels veer out of control.

Saturated fat (animal fat) in the diet is the main factor raising blood levels of cholesterol.

- Cholesterol travels through the bloodstream packaged in lipoproteins.

  Cholesterol carried by low-density lipoprotein (LDL cholesterol) plays a major role in atherosclerotic plaque formation and is called "bad" cholesterol.

  Cholesterol carried by high-density lipoprotein (HDL cholesterol) is known as "good" cholesterol because high levels are associated with a lower risk of heart disease.

  Cholesterol is a lipid, so abnormal levels of the various types of cholesterol are referred to as *dyslipidemias.*

- There is a firm connection between cholesterol levels and heart disease in both men and women.

  The higher your cholesterol levels, the greater your risk.

  The earlier you start controlling your cholesterol levels, the better, whether you have heart disease or not.

CHAPTER
THREE

# Guidelines for Managing Your Cholesterol

O ne organization—and it's a mouthful—the National Cholesterol Education Program (NCEP) Adult Treatment Panel II (ATP II)—has established guidelines for managing high cholesterol.[1] The latest guidelines were released in 1993.

## NCEP Guidelines

If you do not have heart disease, you're one of the fortunate people who has a good chance to prevent any further progression and perhaps never have to face a heart attack or stroke. There's good news also if you currently have heart disease, even if you have already had a heart attack or stroke: You can significantly reduce your chances of another heart attack or stroke and halt or perhaps even reverse further disease progression by following recommended prevention guidelines.

If you're 20 years or older, the guidelines recommend that you have total cholesterol and HDL cholesterol measured at least every 5 years. If you are free of heart disease, a total cholesterol level below 200 mg/dL is considered desirable; 200 to 239 is borderline-high; 240 or above is high. Additionally, an HDL cholesterol level below 35 mg/dL is classified as low. This is good cholesterol, so you want as much of it as possible. (See table 1, NCEP Cholesterol Guidelines in Primary Prevention.) People with heart disease should aim at even lower cholesterol levels.

NCEP risk factors include age, smoking, diabetes, family history, low HDL cholesterol, and high blood pressure. (See table 2, NCEP Risk Factors for Heart Disease.) Obesity, a serious risk factor, is notably missing from the list. Why? Because it affects heart disease through other listed risk factors, such as high blood pressure, diabetes, and low HDL cholesterol.

Since LDL cholesterol (rather than total cholesterol) is most closely associated with increased risk, the decision to start dietary therapy or drug treatment is usually based on it. (See table 3, NCEP Therapy Guidelines Based on LDL

## Table 1. NCEP Cholesterol Guidelines in Primary Prevention

| Total Cholesterol Level (mg/dL) | Classification |
|---|---|
| < 200 | Desirable |
| 200 – 239 | Borderline high |
| ≥ 240 | High |

| HDL Cholesterol Level (mg/dL) | Classification |
|---|---|
| < 35 | Low (increased risk) |
| 35 – 59 | Normal or desirable |
| ≥ 60 | High (decreased risk) |

*Note: < (less than), ≥ (greater than or equal to)*

## Bill's Story: High HDL Cholesterol As a Negative Risk Factor

L evels of HDL cholesterol (the good kind) above 60 are con- sidered to be heart-protective and can be counted as a *negative* risk factor. This means that if you have high HDL cho- lesterol, it reduces your risk factors.

For instance, Bill is a 55-year-old man with hypertension (high blood pressure). Ordinarily, Bill would carry two risk fac- tors: gender/age and hypertension (1 + 1 = 2). But his HDL cholesterol measures a high 64 mg/dL. This cancels out one risk factor, so he would be assessed only one risk factor (2 − 1 = 1).

Cholesterol.) According to these recommendations, about 29% of American adults require dietary intervention and 7% may need drug treatment.[2]

Home cholesterol tests are a quick and easy way to de- termine your total cholesterol level. They require just a single drop of blood from a prick of your finger. However, most such tests don't measure LDL cholesterol or other lipid components. Newer devices that also use a finger-stick blood sample give more complete lipid profiles. Pharma- cies that offer a cholesterol management program for their patients use this type of device.

Studies clearly show the benefits of controlling your cholesterol.[3, 4] Even in high-risk men and women with "av- erage" LDL cholesterol levels of 139 mg/dL, a decrease of 28% in LDL cholesterol lowered the risk of heart attack by 25% and stroke by 28%, and reduced the risk of death from all causes. Further lowering of LDL cholesterol appears to bring correspondingly greater benefit. Additionally, each 1% drop in your total cholesterol lowers your risk of heart attack by 2%. Your risk drops even more, up to 4%, for each 1% your HDL cholesterol climbs up the scale.

## Table 2. NCEP Risk Factors for Heart Disease

Age:   Males, ≥ 45 years old

Females, ≥ 55 years old or premature menopause without estrogen replacement

Current cigarette smoking

Diabetes mellitus

Family history of definite heart attack or sudden death before age 55 in male first-degree relative, or before age 65 in female first-degree relative

Low HDL (< 35 mg/dL)

Hypertension (≥ 140/90) or taking antihypertensive medication

Negative risk factor: High HDL cholesterol (≥ 60 mg/dL— may subtract one other risk factor)

*Note: < (less than), ≥ (greater than or equal to)*

## Table 3. NCEP Therapy Guidelines Based on LDL Cholesterol

| Patient Category | Level (mg/dL) to Start *Dietary* Therapy | LDL Cholesterol Goal |
|---|---|---|
| Without heart disease and < 2 risk factors | ≥ 160 | < 160 |
| Without heart disease and ≥ 2 risk factors | ≥ 130 | < 130 |
| With heart disease | > 100 | ≤ 100 |
| **Patient Category** | **Level (mg/dL) to Start *Drug* Treatment** | **LDL Cholesterol Goal** |
| Without heart disease and < 2 risk factors | ≥ 190 | < 160 |
| Without heart disease and ≥ 2 risk factors | ≥ 160 | < 130 |
| With heart disease | > 130 | ≤ 100 |

*Note: < (less than), > (greater than), ≤ (less than or equal to), ≥ (greater than or equal to)*

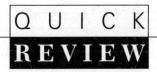

- The National Cholesterol Education Program (NCEP) Adult Treatment Panel II has established guidelines for helping you manage high cholesterol as a key way to prevent heart disease.
- Adhering to recommended prevention guidelines can stall the progression of heart disease and perhaps even coax its retreat.
- If you don't have heart disease, you should keep your total cholesterol and HDL cholesterol below 200 mg/dL and above 35 mg/dL, respectively.
- Generally, the lower your LDL cholesterol, the better. In one study, a 28% reduction in LDL cholesterol significantly diminished the risk of heart attack and stroke. Furthermore, each 1% drop in your total cholesterol lowers your risk of heart attack by 2% and each 1% climb in your HDL cholesterol cuts your risk by as much as 4%.

# Conventional Therapies for High Cholesterol

T he best treatment for heart disease is prevention. If you already have heart disease, there's a lot you can do to stall its progression and protect yourself against heart attack or stroke. One of the most important steps you can take is getting control of your cholesterol levels. In chapters 5 through 7, we will learn about herbs and supplements that can help. But first we will start with the cornerstone of heart disease prevention: a healthful diet and lifestyle.

## Diet and Lifestyle: Your Best Defense Against High Cholesterol

Half of all Americans still have total cholesterol levels that are too high (over 200 mg/dL). The new guidelines urge more aggressive action against high cholesterol, and diet and lifestyle changes are your first-line defense.

Heart-smart dietary and lifestyle choices also protect you against cancer, second only to heart disease as the nation's top killer. Better eating habits, quitting smoking, losing weight, and exercising are the sharpest arrows in your quiver when it comes to fighting heart disease. If you have established heart disease, drugs and other interventions should always be considered additions to dietary and lifestyle changes.

**Half of all Americans still have total cholesterol levels that are too high.**

You may be among the many people who can manage their cholesterol without drugs, simply by focusing on diet, lifestyle, and the selective use of natural agents. We'll look at the latest exciting research on natural agents starting in the next chapter.

## Diet

A balanced diet is the anchor that secures your preventive efforts against high cholesterol and heart disease.[1] Though it requires some effort to change your eating habits, it may help to know that the changes are not as drastic as you might think.

The American Heart Association (AHA) urges you to eat a variety of foods as part of a balanced diet. Adopt eating habits that fit your own lifestyle and that supply the calories, protein, essential fatty acids, carbohydrates, vitamins, minerals, and fiber you need for good health. The best way to do this is to eat foods from all the food groups (See The Food Guide Pyramid later in this chapter). Vitamin and mineral supplements are not a substitute for a balanced and nutritious diet emphasizing fruits, vegetables, and whole-grain foods. Such a diet also helps you avoid excessive calories, sugar, and salt. (See table 4, American Heart Association Step I and Step II Diets.)

## Table 4. American Heart Association
## Step I and Step II Diets

| Dietary Component | Step I Diet | Step II Diet |
|---|---|---|
| Total fat | 30% or less* | 30% or less |
| Saturated Fatty Acids | 8 to 10% | less than 7% |
| Polyunsaturated Fatty Acids | up to 10% | up to 10% |
| Monounsaturated Fatty Acids | up to 15% | up to 15% |
| Carbohydrates | 55% or more | 55% or more |
| Protein | approximately 15% | approximately 15% |
| Cholesterol | less than 300 mg daily | less than 200 mg daily |
| Total Calories | to achieve/maintain desired weight | to achieve/maintain desired weight |

*Note: Percentages refer to percent of total calories (see the Nutrition Facts Food Label discussion)*

## Cutting Back on Fat: How Much?

Of the total calories in the typical American diet, fat makes up between 34 to 40%. According to the experts, this is too much. So how much should you cut back on fat?

In 1993, Dean Ornish, M.D., raised a stir by reporting in the medical journal *Lancet* that a very strict treatment program of diet and lifestyle changes could actually reverse heart disease.[2] To prove it, he put 28 people with heart disease on the following intense regimen:

- A vegetarian diet containing less than 10% total fat and with minimal saturated fat (called the "Reversal Diet").

- Moderate aerobic exercise, usually a walking program.
- Daily stress-management techniques such as stretching, breathing, meditation, yoga, and relaxation exercises.
- Group support and psychological counseling to identify and relieve stress.
- A smoking cessation program for smokers.

For comparison, a "usual care" group of 20 heart disease patients was asked to follow a more conventional diet such as the American Heart Association Step II diet consisting of 30% or less fat and 200 mg of cholesterol daily. They were not asked to make other lifestyle changes, but were free to do so.

The results for the patients on the intensive regimen were impressive to say the least. After 1 year, their LDL-cholesterol dropped 37.2%, they had fewer episodes of angina (chest pain), and their blood vessels showed slightly less blockage. In contrast, the usual care patients showed only a 6% drop in LDL-cholesterol, had more frequent chest pain, and their blood vessels showed slightly more blockage.

But the best was yet to come for the 20 people who had stayed with the intensive regimen. After 5 years, angiograms were used to check the condition of their blood vessels. Researchers found that the blockage in their vessels had actually gone into reverse, *decreasing* by 7.9% (compared to 4.5% after 1 year); again, in contrast, the blockage in the vessels of the 15 people who had stayed with the usual care regimen got much worse, *increasing* by 27.7% (compared to 5.4% after 1 year). Additionally, patients in the usual care group suffered twice as many cardiac events such as heart attack, angioplasty, bypass surgery, and death.

Another interesting finding concerned LDL-cholesterol levels. None of the intensive regimen patients took lipid-lowering drugs. Yet the reduction in their LDL-cholesterol levels was similar to that in the more than half of usual care patients who had been taking lipid-lowering drugs.

In summary, over the course of 5 years, patients on the strict regimen experienced a progressive reversal of their heart disease, while usual care patients got progressively worse.

As a mild counterpoint to the results of the Ornish studies, a recent year-long study of 444 men with high cholesterol suggested you may reach a point of diminishing returns in fat restriction.[3] Researchers found that a moderately fat-restricted diet, such as the AHA diets recommending 30% or less total fat, "attains meaningful and sustained LDL cholesterol reductions." More extreme fat restriction offered little further advantage, and in some cases could have negative effects—such as lowering good cholesterol (HDL cholesterol) and raising triglycerides. However, not all experts agree. Additionally, this study lasted only 1 year and did not look at how the results affected heart disease, as Ornish's groundbreaking studies did.

Ornish's work involved limited number of patients but does indicate that a strict, holistic regimen may reverse lesion progression in heart disease. But it is a rather demanding program. The most difficult part is probably the strict diet, which requires much effort from patient and family. If you are particularly motivated, or if the AHA Step II diet combined with an appropriate exercise program does not bring the results you need, a more strict approach such as that recommended by Ornish may be well worth trying.

## Bad Fat, Good Fat

Fats are present in both animals and plants. Like cholesterol, fat is a type of lipid. The terms *fats* and *fatty acids* are often used interchangeably. The three types of fats are saturated, polyunsaturated, and monounsaturated. Fats actually

## Step I and Step II Diets

The goal of diet therapy is to reduce the risk of heart disease and its consequences such as heart attack. The Step I and Step II diets for the treatment of high blood cholesterol are recommended by the AHA and the National Cholesterol Education Program (NCEP). (See table 4, American Heart Association Step I and Step II Diets.)

The Step I diet is the first step in treating high cholesterol if you don't have established heart disease. If you have heart disease or can't reach your desired cholesterol goal with the Step I diet, you should move to the Step II diet. Start with the Step II diet if your cholesterol level is in the high risk range

consist of a mixture of the three types, and are categorized according to which type is predominant.

- *Saturated* fats include animal fats (beef, pork, and lamb), butter, cream, cream cheese, mayonnaise, salad dressings, coconut and palm oils, and most shortenings (hydrogenated oils).
- *Polyunsaturated* fats include most margarines, vegetable oils (corn, safflower, sunflower, soybean, sesame, and flaxseed), and seeds (flaxseed, sesame, sunflower, and pumpkin).
- *Monounsaturated* fats include olive oil (the most monounsaturated), canola oil, peanut oil, avocado oil, and some margarines.

Saturated fat is the primary fat villain in the heart disease story. The AHA recommends that people's current average intake of saturated fat (12 to 14% of calories) be reduced to

(240 mg/dL and higher) or if you've had a heart attack. If you're overweight, you should combine the diet with regular physical activity and weight reduction. You should also limit your consumption of sugar, salt, and alcohol.

Before the new food label came out, you had to look up foods in a reference guide and make calculations to determine the number of fat calories and grams you were getting. The new food label does this for you, so it's easier than ever before to be aware of what you're doing. (See the Nutrition Facts Food Label discussion later in this chapter.)

that recommended by the Step diets. *Foods high in saturated fats can raise blood cholesterol levels more than anything else you eat, including lowfat, high-cholesterol foods like eggs.*[4]

Substituting polyunsaturated fats or monounsaturated fats for saturated fats appears to be good advice. Saturated fats raise cholesterol levels, but these other fats appear to lower them. However, there is considerable dispute about which is better: polyunsaturated or monounsaturated fats, with neither a clear winner.[5]

Both types of fat significantly lower cholesterol levels. Monounsaturated fats, however, may also raise levels of HDL cholesterol—the good kind.[6]

### Monounsaturated Fats

Monounsaturated fats may offer other advantages. Population studies suggest that olive oil may have protective effects against several cancers, including breast cancer.[7]

## What About Eggs?

For decades we were urged not to eat eggs because they were "high in cholesterol and could clog our arteries," even though they are relatively low in fat. Then it was decided eggs could go back on most menus because dietary cholesterol is less a concern than saturated fat. But if you eat enough dietary cholesterol it may become a problem, so don't go overboard on eggs or any other high-cholesterol food.[8]

Extra-virgin and virgin olive oils are the highest quality, made from first pressing the olives without added chemicals, but less expensive olive oils still appear to be better than many other oils.

Compared to polyunsaturated fats, monounsaturated fats are less prone to oxidize and conjure up damaging free radicals, which are believed to promote heart disease and cancer. In particular, monounsaturated fats hold up better than polyunsaturated fats to heat. Heating speeds oxidation and the production of free radicals.

Olive oil and canola oil seem to be the best oils for cooking. They are composed mainly of oleic acid, a monounsaturated oil more resistant to heat and light than highly polyunsaturated oils. Peanut oil may be a good choice for deep frying, and olive oil can be used in sautéing in place of butter or margarine. Once heated, oils should not be reused, because that can cause further oxidation.

### Polyunsaturated Fats

Omega-3 polyunsaturated fatty acids, the type found primarily in fish, are often recommended because they may have special beneficial effects.[9] However, the evidence for such benefits with fish oil is mixed, with some studies showing none.

Margarine, made of polyunsaturated vegetable oils, was once seen as a safe alternative to butter for lowering cholesterol, but this idea has lost some luster. Margarine is manufactured using a process called *hydrogenation,* which converts some polyunsaturates into saturated fat. This process produces *trans-fatty acids*, which are associated with higher cholesterol levels and, theoretically, with cancer.[10]

The soft-tub form of margarine may be preferable, because it's low in trans-fatty acids. U.S. manufacturers are not presently required to list trans-fats on food product labels.[11] You might achieve an even larger risk reduction by replacing butter and other hard fats with modern low-saturated "zero-trans" margarines, which have a fatty-acid composition approximating that of liquid oils. Recently, special forms of margarine (including one from Finland) have been touted as lowering cholesterol. See chapter 7 for a discussion of a new type of margarine containing the promising cholesterol-lowering plant substance called *sitostanol*.

## Fiber: What You Can't Digest Can Be Good for You

Fiber, sometimes called roughage, creates bulk in the intestines. Fiber is found only in plant foods like whole-grain breads and cereals, beans and peas, and other vegetables and fruits. It's the indigestible structural part of plants, such as celery strings, corn-kernel skins, the membrane sections of an orange, and the bran that surrounds grains.

The AHA recommends 25 to 30 g of dietary fiber a day, but most Americans get only about 10 g. This may be one of the reasons that the Chinese, who consume much higher levels of fiber, have a lower incidence of heart disease than Americans.

There are two types of fiber: soluble and insoluble. Water-soluble fiber can lower blood cholesterol. This type of fiber is found in oat bran, rice bran, psyllium, barley, guar gum, pectin, and cooked dried beans.[12] Insoluble fiber, which appears to provide the best protection against colon cancer, is found in wheat bran and the woody parts of fruits and vegetables.[13]

Many forms of cholesterol-lowering soluble fiber supplements are available, ranging from oat bran to expensive fiber products sold through multilevel marketing firms. The popular press has written extensively about oat bran and psyllium. A good dose of oat bran is 5 to 10 g with each meal and at bedtime; for psyllium, 10 g with each meal. The Food and Drug Administration allows certain psyllium products to state on the label that they can help reduce heart disease risk. However, eating a diet high in fresh fruits and vegetables and whole grains may be even better, because of the many healthful nutrients in such a diet.

## Understanding the Dietary Fat and Fiber Connection

You need a certain amount of dietary fat for good health—it supplies energy, essential fatty acids, and aids absorption of the fat-soluble vitamins A, D, E, and K. However, both heart disease and cancer are related to consuming *too much* fat. Typical high-fat foods such as ice cream, cheese, oils, and non-lean red meats are also low in fiber. The combination of high-fat and low-fiber appears to be worse than either alone.

**The combination of high-fat and low-fiber appears to be worse than either alone.**

Additionally, eating high-fat foods tends to elbow out high-fiber foods—you have room to eat only so much. In fact, a Harvard study reported in the February 14, 1996 issue of the *Journal of the American Medical Association* found that the connection between saturated fat and heart attack is

partially due to lower fiber intake among the men who consumed more fat.[14]

## The Food Guide Pyramid:
## Your Map to Healthful Eating

The Food Guide Pyramid, which replaced the earlier Basic Four Food Groups, is a useful tool devised by the United
States Department of Agriculture (USDA). One of its purposes is to steer you away from diets high in fat toward
nutritionally balanced meals that contain more complex
carbohydrates (starch and fiber).

The Food Guide Pyramid (see figure 1) divides foods
into six groups ranked on four levels, with a recommended
number of daily servings from each group. Here's how it's
arranged, starting from the base:

- Level one consists of the bread, cereal, pasta, and
  rice group.
- Level two consists of the vegetables and fruits group.
- Level three consists of the milk, yogurt, cheese
  group and the meat, poultry, fish, dry beans, eggs,
  nuts group.
- Level four, at the top, consists of the fats, oils, and
  sweets group.

Though dry beans (such as pinto, navy, kidney, and black
beans) are included in the meat and beans group as meat
alternatives, they can also count as vegetables.

In the pyramid, the most important foods are those clos-
est to the base and taking up the largest area in the
illustration. As you can see, you should choose most of your
foods from the grain products group (6 to 11 servings), the
vegetable group (3 to 5 servings), and the fruit group (2 to
4 servings). Try to get at least the minimum number of servings from each group daily.

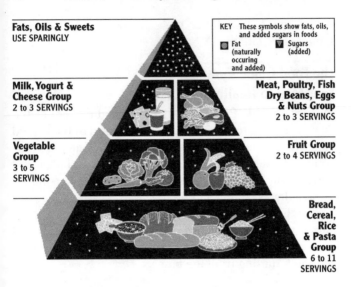

**Figure 1.** *The Food Guide Pyramid*

Eat moderate amounts from the milk group (2 to 3 servings) and the meat and beans group (2 to 3 servings).

Eat sparing amounts from the fats and sweets group at the top—they provide few nutrients and are relatively high in fat and sugars (fats and sugars also occur naturally in the other food groups).

The number of servings from each group varies according to the total calories in your diet. The smaller number of servings in each category is for people consuming about 1,600 calories a day, and the larger number is for those consuming about 2,800 calories a day.

You'll find high-fat foods in the fats and oils group, of course, but you'll also find them in the milk–dairy group, meat–eggs–beans group, and in some processed foods in the bread–grains group. Use the Nutrition Facts Food Label (see the following topic) to help you select foods low in total fat, saturated fat, and cholesterol and higher in fiber. Saturated fat should make up less than 10% of calories (about 20 g per 2,000 calories), and dietary cholesterol should be held below 300 mg daily. Children under age two need a higher percentage of fat calories than adults.

The milk–dairy group provides most of the calcium in the American diet, as well as vitamin D. To secure the benefits and bypass the fat hazard, choose skim or lowfat milk and nonfat yogurt.

**Children under age two need a higher percentage of fat calories than adults.**

## The Nutrition Facts Food Label: Help at the Grocery Store

The USDA's Nutrition Facts food label is a boon for health-conscious consumers (see figure 2). The label enables you to select health-smart foods that will help ward of heart disease as well as cancer and other diseases. It's required on most packaged foods, but not on certain ready-to-eat foods like unpackaged deli and bakery items and restaurant food. Labels are also voluntary for many raw foods, such as fish, meat, poultry, and raw fruits and vegetables that are most frequently consumed.

All manufacturers are required to use the same label format. Once you familiarize yourself with the label, it's easy to use. It clearly states the serving size (in both household and metric measures), number of servings per container, and the number of calories per serving. But that's just the beginning.

For example, the label in figure 2 details the nutrition facts for a package of cookies. The bold line across the middle

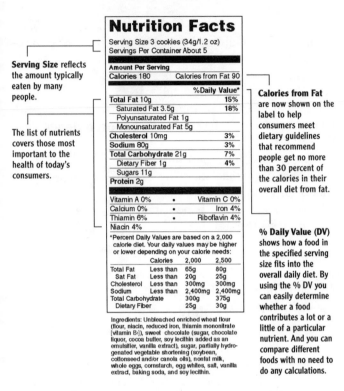

Serving Size reflects the amount typically eaten by many people.

The list of nutrients covers those most important to the health of today's consumers.

**Nutrition Facts**

Serving Size 3 cookies (34g/1.2 oz)
Servings Per Container About 5

**Amount Per Serving**

| Calories 180 | Calories from Fat 90 |
| --- | --- |

| | %Daily Value* |
| --- | --- |
| **Total Fat** 10g | 15% |
| Saturated Fat 3.5g | 18% |
| Polyunsaturated Fat 1g | |
| Monounsaturated Fat 5g | |
| **Cholesterol** 10mg | 3% |
| **Sodium** 80g | 3% |
| **Total Carbohydrate** 21g | 7% |
| Dietary Fiber 1g | 4% |
| Sugars 11g | |
| **Protein** 2g | |

| | | | |
| --- | --- | --- | --- |
| Vitamin A 0% | • | Vitamin C 0% |
| Calcium 0% | • | Iron 4% |
| Thiamin 6% | • | Riboflavin 4% |
| Niacin 4% | | |

*Percent Daily Values are based on a 2,000 calorie diet. Your daily values may be higher or lower depending on your calorie needs:

| | | Calories | 2,000 | 2,500 |
| --- | --- | --- | --- | --- |
| Total Fat | Less than | | 65g | 80g |
| Sat Fat | Less than | | 20g | 25g |
| Cholesterol | Less than | | 300mg | 300mg |
| Sodium | Less than | | 2,400mg | 2,400mg |
| Total Carbohydrate | | | 300g | 375g |
| Dietary Fiber | | | 25g | 30g |

Ingredients: Unbleached enriched wheat flour (flour, niacin, reduced iron, thiamin mononitrate [vitamin B₁], sweet chocolate (sugar, chocolate liquor, cocoa butter, soy lecithin added as an emulsifier, vanilla extract), sugar, partially hydrogenated vegetable shortening (soybean, cottonseed and/or canola oils), nonfat milk, whole eggs, cornstarch, egg whites, salt, vanilla extract, baking soda, and soy lecithin.

**Calories from Fat** are now shown on the label to help consumers meet dietary guidelines that recommend people get no more than 30 percent of the calories in their overall diet from fat.

**% Daily Value (DV)** shows how a food in the specified serving size fits into the overall daily diet. By using the % DV you can easily determine whether a food contributes a lot or a little of a particular nutrient. And you can compare different foods with no need to do any calculations.

**Figure 2.** *The Nutrition Facts Food Label*

divides it into two parts. The top part tells you what's in an individual serving of that product. The first line states that one serving size (three cookies) contains 180 calories, 90 of which are calories from fat. Next comes key information on the food components most associated with maintaining good health—fat (total and saturated), cholesterol, sodium, carbohydrates (including fiber and sugars), and protein.

Let's look at fat content. An individual serving of cookies provides 10 g of total fat, which is 15% of the recommended total daily value (amount). Most dietary guidelines recommend that you get no more than 30% of total daily calories from fat. (The math is done for you. The label is standardized to a 2,000-calorie diet, and 30% of 2,000 calories is 600 calories. Each gram of fat has 9 calories, so 600 divided by 9 is approximately 65 g. The amount of fat in a serving of this product, 10 g, is 15% of 65 g.)

Now look at the lower half of the label, below the information on vitamins, and you'll see columns in smaller print. This is the reference section. The numbers it shows are the same on all food labels—it's there as a reminder for you. These numbers are the total daily values (amounts) associated with a 2,000-calorie diet and a 2,500-calorie diet. The 2,000 column shows 65 g of total fat.

**Egg whites do not contain cholesterol.**

Though information is listed for a 2,500-calorie diet, the individual serving information in the top half of the label is based on a 2,000-calorie diet. If you are on a diet with fewer than 2,000 calories or more than 2,500 calories, you may have to do a bit figuring yourself. However, once you become accustomed to the label, you'll be able to estimate fairly closely for other caloric amounts.

The last item at the bottom of the label tells you the number of calories per gram of fat (9), carbohydrates (4), and protein (4). As you can see, fat is the highest source of dietary calories. The bottom line: If you eat those three cookies, you've consumed 15% of the recommended allotted fat intake for the day (if you're on a 2,000-calorie diet). The fat can add up fast. Some experts think that the 30% target is too high and recommend getting less than 20% of daily calories from fat.

## Tips to Trim Dietary Fats

The USDA has determined that the average person eats about 20 food items a day. To stay on target, your fat intake should average 5% per food item (5% x 20 = 100%), though you will go above or below the average on individual products.

Here are some more ways to trim fats from your diet:

1. Eat lowfat, low-cholesterol foods, as recommended by the American Heart Association:
   - Fruits and vegetables
   - Whole grains like cereal, rice, and pasta
   - Lean red meats and poultry without skin
   - Lowfat or skim-milk dairy products
   - Lean fish and shellfish
   - Beans and peas
   - Nuts and seeds in limited amounts
   - Unsaturated vegetable oils like olive, canola, safflower, and sunflower oils (in limited amounts)

2. Become familiar with the Nutrition Facts food label and consult it when purchasing foods.
   - *Fats and oils group:* Use small amounts of high-fat salad dressings and spreads such as butter, margarine, and mayonnaise. Use lowfat or fat-free dressings for salads,

## Exercise: Strengthen Your Heart and Body

Physical inactivity is a welcome mat for heart disease and death from it.[15] Regular exercise or activity—especially the aerobic type—can jerk away the welcome mat and replace it with a "No Vacancy" sign. Your exercise capacity will increase or no dressings at all. Use less butter, margarine, and oils (cooking oils, salad dressings, and so on) Use olive oil for cooking and salad dressings. Cut out or use less mayonnaise or similar dressings on sandwiches.

- *Bread–grains, vegetables, and fruits group:* Eat lowfat sauces with pasta, rice, and potatoes. Use minimal fats and oils in cooking vegetables and grain products. For seasoning, use spices, herbs, lemon juice, and lowfat or fat-free salad dressings.

- *Meat–eggs–beans group:* Eat less red meat—substitute chicken and fish instead. Select meats labeled "lean" or "extra lean." Trimming visible fat from meat and removing skin from poultry can cut fat by up to half. Most beans are lowfat and good sources of fiber and protein. Reduce your intake of processed meats and cold cuts. If you eat these, use the Nutrition Facts label to compare fat grams. Limit organ meats and egg yolks, which tend to be high in cholesterol (egg whites do not contain cholesterol). Broil, roast, or poach meats and drain off fat after cooking.

- *Milk–dairy group:* Use skim or lowfat milk, lowfat or fat-free yogurt, and lowfat cheese.

and your risk of heart disease will drop.[16] You'll get and keep these benefits at any level of regular physical activity, whether you're healthy or have heart disease.[17]

Exercise helps, but *how* does it help? Apart from increasing your cardiovascular fitness, physical activity takes the wind out of several risk factors for heart disease. Regular exercise

## Getting Exercise from Everyday Activities

You might think of exercise as something that must be done apart from your daily routine. But studies show that modifying your daily activities to include regular "exercise" also works.[18] If done regularly, the benefits add up. Here are some simple ways you can get these heart-protective benefits:

- Park farther from your destination and walk the rest of the way.
- Take the stairs instead of the escalator or elevator.
- Work in the garden or yard.
- Think of ways to add regular physical activity to your own particular routine.

helps control cholesterol, obesity, and diabetes. Aerobic exercise can also lower your blood pressure (both systolic and diastolic) by 8 to 10 mm Hg in many cases. Moderate-intensity activity is all it takes to get the benefits.[19] A university hospital study of 742 predominantly healthy men found that moderate exercise decreased systolic blood pressure and fasting insulin levels, and both glucose and insulin levels during a 3-hour oral glucose tolerance test.[20] In another study, exercise reduced blood vessel resistance (the force against which your heart must pump). This resistance makes blood pressure climb higher, especially in elderly people. In this way, exercise eases your heart's workload.[21]

A recipe that combines physical activity with other positive ingredients such as stopping smoking, controlling cholesterol, and losing weight has the power to stop the spread of atherosclerotic plaque and in some cases even send it in retreat.[22]

## How Much Exercise Do You Need?

When you think of exercise, do you imagine a sweat-drenched body pushing itself to the max in the weight room or on a treadmill? You don't have to go till you drop, and you don't even have to exercise as "regularly" as you might think to help prevent heart disease and lose weight.

The current thinking by fitness experts is that less can be more. The most obvious reason is that if your exercise regimen is too intense or time-consuming, you may not stick with it. It's estimated that only half of people who start an exercise program will stay with it more than 6 months.[23]

Sticking to a program is critical, because exercise is beneficial only if it's maintained for extended periods of time. Most experts think that the key is to find the type of exercise you enjoy—whether weight training, aerobics, walking, swimming, or sports activities—and the level of exertion that makes you feel good. To sum up, it's not the time or intensity—or even frequency, within reason—of exercising that's most important, but the regularity over the long term.[24]

**It's not the time or intensity—or even frequency, within reason—of exercising that's most important, but the regularity over the long term.**

Try to build up to about 30 minutes a session on a regular basis—at least 3 times a week. Spread it out for the best results, such as every other day. Start slowly and build up gradually as your heart gets stronger.

Before starting an exercise program, check with your physician. If you're inexperienced, you may also want to get advice from an exercise specialist. See the sidebar, Getting

## Exercise and Your Target Heart Rate

Some exercise specialists recommend maintaining your "target heart rate" for a continuous period of time during exercise to get the most benefit. Here's how to figure your target heart rate:

1. Subtract your age from 220—this is your predicted maximal heart rate (heartbeats per minute).
2. Multiply the result by 0.65 and then 0.80 to get your target heart rate range.

If you're 40 years old, for example, during exercise you want to stay within the range of 117 to 144 heartbeats a minute. Here's how that was figured:

$$220 - 40 = 180$$
$$180 \times 0.65 = 117$$
$$180 \times 0.80 = 144$$

Exercise from Everyday Activities for hints on informal exercise alternatives.

## Body Weight: Avoid Unneeded Baggage

Burdening your body with extra pounds undermines your health in numerous ways. Getting to a healthy weight and staying there improves blood cholesterol levels and blood pressure and significantly lowers your risk of heart disease and stroke, as well as certain cancers.[25] The road to a desirable weight is paved with a combination of regular physical activity and a diet limited in calories, especially those from fat, and rich in complex carbohydrates and fiber.[26]

If you carry too much fat around the midsection, dropping even a few pounds lowers both triglycerides and small, dense LDL cholesterol, while raising your HDL cholesterol. Losing weight also decreases the insulin resistance associated with diabetes.[27]

Body mass index (BMI) is a way to compare weight to height. A desirable weight means having a BMI of 21 to 25. For example, a healthy weight for a person who is 5' 9" would be 142 to 168 pounds—with the higher end of the scale applying to people with more muscle and bone.[28] The less active you are, the lower your BMI should be. This guideline is similar to that of a federal task force, which considers an ideal BMI to be 19 to 25. Values greater than 25 are associated with obesity and values lower than 18.5 reflect malnutrition. For individuals over 65, an ideal BMI may be about 27.

BMI is not a perfect standard, however. The index does not reflect body composition—for instance, a very muscular individual may have a high BMI but a low body-fat percentage.

## Smoking: Find a Way to Beat It Before It Beats You

Plain and simple, smoking is a lightning rod for heart disease. The best advice is the bluntest: Stop smoking as soon as you can. Good things start to happen in your body soon after you tamp out that last cigarette. Consider the following timetable of beneficial health changes you may expect to occur after quitting:

**A smoker's risk of heart attack is more than twice that of nonsmokers.**

- IN 20 MINUTES: Your blood pressure falls and your pulse rate returns to normal.

## How to Calculate Your Body Mass Index (BMI)

The BMI is the number derived from your weight in kilograms divided by your height in meters squared. For example, if you weigh 150 lb and you're 5' 6" (66 inches) tall:

150 divided by 2.2 = 68.2 kg
(66 multiplied by 2.54) divided by 100 = 1.68 m
1.68 squared (i.e., 1.68 x 1.68) = 2.8
68.2 divided by 2.8 = BMI 24.4

- IN 24 HOURS: Your chance of an immediate heart attack diminishes.
- IN 48 HOURS: Your taste and smell are enhanced.
- IN 2 WEEKS TO 3 MONTHS: Your blood circulation improves and your lung function increases up to 30%.
- IN 1 MONTH TO 9 MONTHS: Coughing, sinus congestion, fatigue, and shortness of breath decrease. Your lung function continues to improve and overall energy increases.
- IN 1 YEAR: Your risk of heart disease is now half that of a smoker.
- IN 5 YEARS: Your risk of death from lung cancer drops by almost half. In 5 to 15 years after quitting, your risk of stroke is reduced to that of a nonsmoker. Your risk of cancer of the mouth and throat is half that of a smoker.
- IN 10 YEARS: Your risk of death from lung cancer is similar to a nonsmoker.
- IN 15 YEARS: Your risk of heart disease is the same as a nonsmoker.

Smoking is such a huge risk factor for heart disease that the Surgeon General has called it "the most important of the known modifiable risk factors for coronary heart disease in the United States." And you probably don't need to be reminded that smoking is also an open invitation to cancer.

According to the AHA, a smoker's risk of heart attack is more than twice that of nonsmokers. In fact, cigarette smoking is the risk factor most associated with sudden cardiac death. Smokers who suffer a heart attack are more likely to die and die suddenly (within an hour) than nonsmokers. Evidence also suggests that passive smoking (chronic exposure to tobacco smoke) may increase the risk of heart disease. If you need help quitting, check with a local hospital about available smoking cessation resources. A program might include nicotine replacement therapy and/or the prescription drug bupropion.

**The best advice is the bluntest: Stop smoking as soon as you can. Good things start to happen in your body soon after you tamp out that last cigarette.**

## Alcohol: Less May Be More

Though studies suggest that moderate alcohol (ethanol) intake may lower the risk of heart disease,[29] the AHA generally discourages its consumption because of the dangers associated with excessive use, such as alcoholism, hypertension, obesity, stroke, liver disease, and cancer, as well as the danger of accidents.

The American Cancer Society also discourages alcohol use, but acknowledges that moderate intake—two drinks a day for men and one for women—appears to lower the risk of heart disease in middle-aged adults. However, the ACS says, women at unusually high risk for breast cancer may wish to consider abstaining from alcohol altogether. A drink is typically defined as 12 ounces of beer, 5 ounces of wine, or 1.5 ounces of 80-proof liquor.[30]

The cardiovascular benefits of drinking a glass or two of red wine a day have been well documented. Recently, an international symposium of experts concluded that drinking moderate amounts of white wine, beer, and liquor was just as effective as red wine in reducing the risk of coronary heart disease in older people.[31] Older, high-risk people who drink one to three bottles of beer, glasses of wine, or shots of hard liquor are 25% less likely to suffer heart disease and stroke than nondrinkers.

Be aware: Amounts higher than the equivalent of about two drinks per day of any kind of alcohol is associated with an increased risk of infarction and stroke.

## What About Coffee?

If you like to drink coffee in moderate amounts, there seems to be no clear reason to stop. Some studies have found that drinking coffee may increase cardiovascular risk slightly.[32] However, other studies show no effect of coffee when other factors such as smoking and high intake of saturated fat are taken into account.[33]

## What Are Lipid-Lowering Drugs?

An intensive nondrug approach can substantially lower your cholesterol—if you're willing to devote the effort to it.

However, if you need to lower your LDL cholesterol by 25% or more, you may need drug therapy.[34]

Your foremost therapy goal is getting your LDL cholesterol under 100 mg/dL. You also want to boost your HDL cholesterol level above 35 mg/dL and push down your triglycerides below 200 mg/dL.

Your doctor will consider drug therapy in addition to diet and exercise when these lifestyle changes alone don't do the job, or when your risk of immediate cardiac complications is high. For guidelines on when to start drug therapy in people with and without heart disease, see table 3 in chapter 3, NCEP Therapy Guidelines Based on LDL Cholesterol.

## Statins (HMG-CoA Reductase Inhibitors)

Statin drugs have become the most widely used lipid-lowering drugs. They include lovastatin (Mevacor), pravastatin (Pravachol), simvastatin (Zocor), fluvastatin (Lescol), atorvastatin (Lipitor), and cerivastatin (Baycol). Lovastatin, the first statin, was introduced in 1987, the same year that the National Cholesterol Education Program (NCEP) released its first guidelines.

Statins lower LDL cholesterol by muzzling an enzyme called HMG CoA reductase. This blocks a key step in the liver's manufacture of very-low-density lipoprotein (VLDL). VLDL is converted to LDL cholesterol.[35] The liver reacts by removing LDL cholesterol from the bloodstream to restore the cholesterol that was lost due to reduced production of VLDL. The result is a fall in LDL cholesterol blood levels.

The drugs lower LDL cholesterol by 20 to 61% and triglycerides by 10 to 37%, and increase HDL cholesterol by 2 to 12%. Atorvastatin appears to be especially effective in reducing both LDL cholesterol and triglycerides.

Numerous well-designed clinical trials have demonstrated the ability of statins to lower LDL cholesterol levels and reduce both deaths from heart disease and deaths from other causes in people with heart disease. Let's briefly look at a couple of them.

The Scandinavian Simvastatin Survival Study (4S) was the first to link lipid-lowering therapy with a decrease in deaths from all causes. It followed 4,444 men and women with a history of angina or heart attack over 5.4 years.[36] Participants who took simvastatin showed decreases of 25%, 35%, and 10% in total cholesterol, LDL cholesterol, and triglycerides, respectively; HDL cholesterol increased by 8%. The average LDL cholesterol level fell from 188 mg/dL to 122 mg/dL. The number of heart attacks and strokes declined, as well as total deaths and the need for bypass and angioplasty procedures. There was no increase in non-cardiac deaths, an important finding that provided reassurance that statins were safer than some other forms of lipid-lowering therapy in this regard.

The Cholesterol and Recurrent Events (CARE) Trial showed that pravastatin could reduce the risk of recurrent cardiac events even in survivors of acute heart attack with "average" LDL-cholesterol levels of 139 mg/dL. It followed 4,158 men and women with a history of recent heart attack for 5 years.[37] The patient mix included smokers and those with high blood pressure or diabetes; 54% had a history of bypass or angioplasty procedures. In the drug group, LDL cholesterol fell by 28%, heart attacks by 25%, and strokes by 28%. The benefits were not affected by high blood pressure, diabetes, smoking, or heart failure.

Side effects of statins include reversible liver enzyme elevations, gastrointestinal upset, headache, dizziness, mild skin rashes, muscle pain, and, rarely, muscle inflammation at high doses. In most cases, you should not take statins if you have elevated liver enzymes, a history of liver disease, or drink significant amounts of alcoholic beverages. Elevated liver enzymes usually return to normal after stopping the drug, but serious liver toxicity is possible. Because of this risk, your liver function should be checked after 6 and 12 weeks of therapy and periodically thereafter. For more information on these medications, see *The Natural Pharmacist Guide to Garlic and Cholesterol.*

## Fibrates

Fibrates include gemfibrozil (Lopid), clofibrate (Atromid-D), and the investigational agents bezafibrate and fenofibrate. They appear to work by activating the enzyme lipoprotein lipase, which results in a triglyceride-lowering effect. They may also lower VLDL.

Gemfibrozil, the fibrate most widely used in the United States, can lower triglycerides by 25 to 40% and increase HDL cholesterol. The downside is that it's prone to send LDL cholesterol up the scale instead of down. This may require a change to another drug or the addition of a second drug. Of the commonly used lipid-lowering drugs, gemfibrozil is least likely to do much for high LDL cholesterol levels.

These drugs are fairly well-tolerated in the short term, with mild gastrointestinal distress as the major side effect. Rarely, hepatitis can occur. Long-term use may be associated with a two-fold increased risk of gallstones. Some doctors are reluctant to use fibrates because of long-term safety concerns. In an analysis of several studies in which fibrates were used, there was a slight increase in overall deaths despite reductions in cardiac events and deaths.

## Bile Acid Sequestrants (Resins)

Resins include cholestyramine (Questran) and colestipol (Colestid). They work by binding bile acids in the intestines and carrying them out of the body. Because the liver needs cholesterol to make more bile acids, it recruits LDL cholesterol from the blood, thus lowering LDL cholesterol

levels. These drugs also increase HDL cholesterol slig
Unfortunately, they may raise triglycerides by up to 1
For that reason, you should not use resins if you have
triglycerides unless you also take a drug that counter
the triglycerides-raising effect. People don't like to
resins because they taste bad, require large doses, and
cause gastrointestinal discomfort.

## Should You Take Estrogen?

You may have heard that estrogen can protect won
against heart disease. Should you take estrogen? Let's
a closer look.

Despite similar risk factors, women in their reprodu
years have a lower risk of heart disease than men. Th
thought to be at least partly due to the protective effect
trogen has on the heart. After menopause, however, estro
levels fall. This puts women at greater risk for heart dise
the leading cause of death in postmenopausal women.

The positive effects of estrogen against heart disease
clude lowering LDL cholesterol, raising HDL cholest
and possible antioxidant effects.[38] A 1998 review of larg
als of estrogen therapy leads the author to conclude that
ERT (estrogen replacement therapy) and HRT (horn
replacement therapy—estrogen plus progestin) significa
protects postmenopausal women against heart disease. H
ever, there are flaws in all these studies, and a report iss
at the time of this writing has somewhat undermined fai
estrogen's protective effects. Furthermore, many women
afraid to use this therapy because of the possible incre
risk of uterine (or endometrial) cancer and breast cance
sociated with it.[39]

In a recent review of a number of studies, the aut
expressed concern about the risk of endometrial cancer

breast cancer associated with estrogen.[40] They advised that, until definitive scientific findings provide solid evidence of the preventive effects of estrogen against heart disease, it should not be recommended routinely for all postmenopausal women.

We know that estrogen therapy helps prevent osteoporosis and colorectal cancer, and, of course, alleviates menopausal symptoms. Most experts still believe that the benefits of estrogen therapy—especially in regard to heart disease—outweigh the risks.

## Angioplasty and Bypass Surgery

What about surgical means to correct heart disease? Percutaneous transluminal coronary angioplasty (PTCA) and coronary artery bypass graft surgery (CABG) are invasive methods used to restore blood flow to the heart lost due to blocked coronary arteries.[41] These procedures should be reserved for people at high-risk who don't respond to other therapy methods.

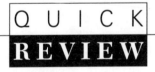

QUICK REVIEW

- Eating better, exercising, losing weight, and quitting smoking should be the pillars supporting your efforts to prevent heart disease.
- New guidelines urge that you keep your cholesterol in tight check. The recommended diet is a lowfat, low-cholesterol diet. This diet should consist primarily of fruits and vegetables, whole grains, and lean meats.

- You should consider drug therapy in addition to diet and exercise:

    When these lifestyle changes alone don't help enough;

    When your cholesterol is too high;

    When your risk of immediate cardiac complications is high.

- Numerous major studies have confirmed the beneficial effects of managing lipid levels.

    The most widely used lipid-lowering drugs are the statins.

- Hormone replacement therapy (HRT) may help protect post-menopausal women against heart disease.

- When standard therapy has failed, some patients may be candidates for angioplasty or bypass surgery.

# Niacin and
# High Cholesterol

**C**onventional and natural therapies for heart disease, once separate, have begun to overlap. The lifestyle practices discussed in the last chapter—eating healthful foods, increasing physical activity, and stopping smoking—should be the underpinnings of your efforts to lower your cholesterol by natural means. These fundamental lifestyle practices not only protect you against heart disease, but also against cancer and other chronic diseases.

In addition, there are specific nutrient and herbal supplements that can lower your cholesterol levels and perhaps protect your heart in other ways. If your cholesterol levels are very high, and your arteries are already in bad condition, it might be wiser to turn to proven drug treatments. However, if your physician says you can safely spend some time exploring other options, the natural therapies described in the following chapters may be worth trying.

Sometimes, your cholesterol may remain high despite your best efforts. If this happens, conventional treatment may be necessary.

## Epidemiologic (Population) Study

An *epidemiologic* study (also called a population or observational study) looks for disease trends in populations. It usually looks at what people did in the past. Participants may fill out surveys or questionnaires on what they recall about particular behaviors, such as what foods they ate or what nutritional supplements they took in past years.

This type of study, by its nature, is open to mixed interpretation. Suppose, for example, such a study found that foods high in vitamin C protect against heart disease. Does this mean that vitamin C supplements protect against heart disease as well? Not necessarily. The protective effect may be due to other nutrients and phytochemicals present in vitamin C–rich foods.

Or suppose that a study found that people who take vitamin E supplements get less heart disease. This seems more airtight until you realize that people who take vitamin E supplements may also be more likely to engage in various healthful lifestyle habits. The question becomes, then, are the results due to the vitamin E supplement or to something else these people do? You can see how tricky things can get.

## Niacin

In the 1950s, high doses of the vitamin niacin were found to lower high cholesterol levels. Niacin has been part of conventional lipid-lowering treatment ever since, and is a good example of the melding of conventional and natural therapies.

The National Cholesterol Education Program (NCEP) considers niacin to be in the same league as the lipid-lowering drugs discussed in chapter 4. NCEP further suggests that niacin is especially valuable in treating high cholesterol in people with low HDL cholesterol, and in people with both high cholesterol and high triglycerides.

Before the statin drugs arrived, niacin was the most commonly prescribed cholesterol-lowering agent. It does have one primary drawback, however: unpleasant side effects.

This over-the-counter vitamin really does work, but you need to be aware of some potential potholes to sidestep. We'll cover everything you need to know to help you take niacin safely.

**Since the 1950s, high doses of niacin have been part of conventional lipid-lowering treatment.**

## What Is Niacin?

Niacin (nicotinic acid) or vitamin $B_3$, is a water-soluble vitamin that was identified in the 1930s as an essential nutrient.[1] As a vitamin, niacin is unusual because the body can manufacture it from the dietary amino acid tryptophan, which is also the precursor of the brain transmitter serotonin. Niacin itself is present in various foods.

Niacinamide, a compound produced by the body's breakdown of niacin, possesses the same vitamin activity but not the cholesterol-lowering properties. Niacinamide is the form used in most multivitamin supplements because it does not cause the flushing side effect of niacin (see Safety Issues, later).

## Clinical Intervention Trial

The *intervention* trial is a more definitive study design. In this type of study, researchers "intervene" in people's lives in some way to see what happens. For instance, participants might take a nutritional supplement thought to help prevent a particular disease. This study follows participants into the future to see if they are less likely to get the disease than others not taking the agent.

These studies are very expensive to perform because they must be continued for many years and enroll high numbers of people. You should give intervention trials the most weight when trying to decide whether a treatment works.

The best type of intervention trial:

■ Uses a *control group* receiving either no treatment or *placebo* (inactive pill).

## What Is the Scientific Evidence for Niacin?

Solid evidence shows niacin works in both people with and without heart disease. In people without heart disease, niacin appears to reduce deaths from heart disease as well as deaths from all causes.[2] In a long-term trial in people with heart disease, niacin significantly reduced the incidence of heart attack. An even longer-term follow-up of that study (15 years total) found an 11% decrease in deaths from all causes among those taking niacin.[3]

Niacin's effect on cholesterol has been extensively studied, in both its regular (immediate-release) and slow-release forms.[4] Although there are some differences between the two forms of niacin in their effects on lipids, the benefits of both are significant. In high doses, niacin lowers both total

- *Randomly* assigns participants to the treatment and control groups.
- Uses the *double-blind* format, in which neither researchers nor subjects know which treatment each participant receives.
- Some trials use the *crossover* method, in which each participant receives both the treatment and the placebo at different times during the trial.

A *meta-analysis* looks at the combined results from a number of selected trials. However, there are many problems in interpreting the results of such overviews, and they aren't regarded as completely reliable.

*Statistical significance* is determined by various mathematical techniques that tell us whether the results of a study are meaningful.

---

cholesterol and LDL cholesterol by 15 to 25% and decreases triglycerides by 20 to 50%. Additionally, it increases HDL cholesterol as much as 15 to 25% (one of the few agents that does this).

## Dosage

The adult daily value of niacin is 19 mg for most adult men and 15 mg for most adult women.[5] Cholesterol-lowering doses are much higher (up to 3,000 mg daily).

As a cholesterol-lowering agent, you should start niacin at a low dose and gradually increase it over several weeks. For example, begin with 50 to 100 mg 3 times daily taken with or just after meals. Increase the dose 100 to 250 mg every 7 to 14 days. Your goal dose would typically be 500 to

1,000 mg 3 times daily. Dosages up to 6 to 9 g have been used, but larger doses carry a greater potential of side effects. Due to the many complicating factors, you should discuss with your physician which would be better for you: regular or slow-release niacin.

**Niacin lowers both total cholesterol and LDL cholesterol by 15 to 25%, decreases triglycerides by 20 to 50%, and raises HDL cholesterol as much as 15 to 25%.**

A special form of niacin, inositol hexaniacinate, called "flushless" niacin, has been developed in Europe.[6] The term flushless is not quite accurate—some people do flush with inositol hexaniacinate, but the flush is not as common or as severe as with traditional niacin. (As you'll read in Safety Issues, slow-release niacin may also partially get around this problem.) As with niacin, monitoring for possible liver toxicity is necessary.

The dose of inositol hexaniacinate is 500 to 1,000 mg 3 times a day, taken with food. The usual recommendation is to start with the lower dose and only raise it if cholesterol doesn't fall sufficiently after about 6 weeks.

Niacin is present in most foods, including lean meats, liver, fish, poultry, whole-grain and enriched breads and cereals, green vegetables, nuts, and legumes. Its precursor tryptophan is found primarily in animal protein.[7] Cholesterol-lowering doses are far higher than you can get from food, however.

## Safety Issues

Niacin is inexpensive and is available over the counter. It has more side effects than the other lipid-lowering agents, and these limit its popularity. The first thing you will notice within 15 minutes to two hours of taking niacin is its most common side effect: a skin reaction called flushing. Knowing in advance that it's not dangerous does not make it any more comfortable. Prepare for your face and body to turn a shade of red, along with heat sensations, tingling, headache, and itching. You may experience one or more of these symptoms.

Other side effects may include nausea, gastrointestinal discomfort, and diarrhea. Dry skin and eyes are also common, and may be alleviated with skin lotions and artificial tears drops. Elevated blood levels of uric acid can occur and may result in gout in people predisposed for it. A rare skin disorder called acanthosis nigricans is also a possibility.

Fortunately, the flushing reaction tends to diminish after several weeks of therapy. You can minimize it by starting niacin at a low dose and gradually increasing it. Taking doses with food may also help. Taking aspirin 30 minutes before each niacin dose may prevent much of the discomfort. Ibuprofen also appears to work. Aspirin and ibuprofen inhibit prostaglandins, body chemicals that appear to play a role in the flushing reaction. One study found that a 325-mg dose of aspirin (one regular aspirin tablet, non-enteric-coated) is adequate to reduce flushing symptoms, and no higher dose is needed.[8]

The slow-release form of niacin was developed to get around the flushing problem of regular niacin. It worked for that, but brought problems of its own—it appears to be harder on the stomach and liver. The liver problem is the most worrisome.[9] It occurs most often at higher doses (over 2,000 mg daily).[10]

The good news is that liver problems are generally mild and go away when you stop taking niacin. However, rare serious consequences have been reported, including one patient who required a liver transplantation. Liver toxicity has appeared after as little as 1 week of therapy to as long

# Carol's Story: Which Form of Niacin Should You Take?

C arol is 56 years old with no history of heart disease. A fasting lipid profile reveals a total cholesterol level of 270 mg/dL. Her HDL cholesterol is 56, her LDL cholesterol 194, and her triglycerides 100.

Next, her doctor determines her risk for heart disease. She has only one risk factor—she is postmenopausal. In this case, the guideline recommends an LDL cholesterol of 160 or lower. Carol's LDL cholesterol is 194, so she needs to lower it by at least 34 points (17.5%).

Since Carol is not at immediate risk for cardiac problems, her doctor gives her the option of reducing her cholesterol through diet and exercise. She has 3 to 6 months to get her cholesterol into the healthy range.

Carol is determined. She tries her best to eat a balanced diet with plenty of fruits and vegetables and fiber, and she walks for at least 20 minutes almost every day.

After 6 months, Carol shows fair improvement—her LDL cholesterol drops from 194 to 177. However, it still needs lowering by at least 10% to reach her goal of 160. That makes her a candidate for drug therapy.

as 48 months. Flu-like symptoms can be a warning sign of liver problems, including malaise, fatigue, weakness, sleepiness, appetite loss, nausea, vomiting, epigastric pain, and dark urine.[11]

Most people on niacin therapy who developed liver problems were found to be taking slow-release niacin, often after

Carol is not fond of the idea of taking drugs, so she asks her doctor if she can try niacin, and he agrees. Niacin is also likely to boost her HDL cholesterol level from 56 to 60 or above, which would cancel out her one risk factor.

The next decision is more difficult: Which form should she take? Carol discusses the pros and cons with her doctor. Since she needs to lower her LDL cholesterol by only 10% or more, either would probably work. Her friend stopped taking regular niacin because of the flushing reaction, but Carol fears the possible liver toxicity that may be more likely to occur with slow-release niacin. She could also try inositol hexaniacinate, a special form of niacin that may minimize flushing. However, it has not been proven as effective or any safer.

Finally, Carol decides to try regular niacin and see if she can manage the flushing reaction. If not, she intends to try the slow-release form at a dose below 2,000 mg, which appears to be easier on the liver and still capable of lowering her LDL cholesterol by at least 10%. She agrees to schedule regular office visits so her doctor can monitor her for side effects.

being switched from the regular form.[12] It must be said that some studies have found few cases of liver toxicity with slow-release niacin.[13] This suggests that differences in various formulations of slow-release niacin might come into play. Still, many different slow-release niacin products have been associated with liver toxicity. It's also been suggested that the problem may be related to a contaminant introduced during the manufacturing process, but there's no supporting evidence for this.

At doses below 2,000 mg (for example, 1,500 mg), slow-release niacin appears to be safer on the liver, and still produces solid, although less dramatic cholesterol-lowering effects.[14]

Because niacin can be hard on the liver, you should not take it if you have active liver disease or a history of liver disease. The same holds true if you consume large amounts of alcohol.

Although niacin works just as well on cholesterol in people with diabetes mellitus, it may raise blood glucose levels and make control of blood glucose more difficult, so use it cautiously if you're in this group.[15]

If you've had peptic ulcers, you should use niacin cautiously or not at all.

Do not combine niacin with other cholesterol-lowering drugs. Disulfiram (Antabuse), a drug used to treat alcoholism, may intensify the flushing side effect of niacin, so avoid this combination.

**Warning:** Don't take niacin in cholesterol-lowering doses without medical supervision. At those high doses, niacin is a drug, not a dietary supplement. While you're on niacin therapy, your doctor will want to periodically check your blood liver enzymes to head off any possible liver toxicity, niacin's most serious potential side effect.

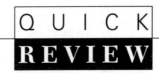

■ Niacin (nicotinic acid) or vitamin $B_3$, is a water-soluble vitamin.

   In high doses, it lowers LDL cholesterol and triglycerides and raises HDL cholesterol.

   Studies have shown that niacin reduces the incidence of heart attack and reduces deaths from heart disease and other causes.

■ Some side effects are associated with niacin.

   The skin reaction called flushing has prevented niacin from becoming a more widely used cholesterol-lowering agent, but there are ways to minimize it.

   A more serious potential problem is liver toxicity, which is associated more often with the slow-release form of niacin.

   Liver problems generally clear up when niacin is stopped.

■ The regular form of niacin is a uniquely effective cholesterol-lowering agent that most people can take safely, provided they undergo careful clinical monitoring. See the chapter for additional safety warnings.

# Garlic and
# High Cholesterol

**G**arlic is the best-documented herbal treatment for high cholesterol. It may also help prevent atherosclerosis in several other ways. For that reason it will appear several times in this book. For more detailed information, see *The Natural Pharmacist Guide to Garlic and Cholesterol.*

## A Brief History of Garlic

Garlic can be found almost everywhere in the world. It has a cult following second only to that of ginseng. Its species name, *sativum,* means "cultivated," which indicates that garlic does not grow in the wild. Since ancient times, peoples of all cultures have used garlic for a wide range of conditions. As far back as the first century A.D., Dioscorides wrote of garlic's ability to "clear the arteries."

In the twentieth century, European medical researchers began to study this ancient herb. As the atherosclerosis–

cholesterol connection became clear, Dioscorides' statement that garlic can clear the arteries finally found a scientific mooring.

As we'll see, there is considerable evidence that garlic can lower cholesterol levels. Garlic also appears to provide other cardiovascular benefits, such as lowering blood pressure and reducing blood clotting.

## What Is in Garlic?

Of the many bioactive compounds in garlic, *allicin* is widely regarded as one of the most important. Others include alliin, ajoene, diallyl disulfide, diallyl trisulfide, s-allyl cysteine, and vinyldithiines. We don't know which of these are the most important.

Little or no allicin exists in an intact garlic bulb. However, when garlic is crushed or cut, an enzyme reaction manufactures allicin out of alliin. Contact with dilute allicin is fatal to a wide variety of bacteria, fungi, viruses, and parasites, so this may be a self-defense mechanism.[1]

**Considerable evidence exists that garlic can lower cholesterol levels.**

The strong odor and irritant properties may also drive away insects. (Legend has it that garlic also repels vampires, but this effect has been observed only among ordinary people in certain social situations.)

Allicin itself is a very unstable compound, and breaks down rapidly once it is formed. This presents a problem to manufacturers who wish to supply an active and yet palatable form of garlic to consumers. Garlic cloves would work, but the smell is too strong for most people. The type of garlic most often used in studies is standardized to contain alliin rather than allicin. That's because alliin has little aroma. The alliin is converted to allicin somewhere in the digestive tract, producing beneficial effects with relatively little odor.

## What Is the Scientific Evidence That Garlic Reduces Cholesterol?

Considerable evidence affirms garlic's cholesterol-lowering abilities.[2] Depending on the study and form of garlic used, the herb may lower total cholesterol by 6 to 12%, LDL cholesterol by 4 to 11%, and triglycerides by 17%. The effects on HDL cholesterol appear to be minimal. These are not gigantic benefits, but they may be all some patients need—such as Carol, whom we met in chapter 5.

**Garlic also appears to provide other cardiovascular benefits, such as lowering blood pressure and reducing blood clotting.**

Many animal studies point to garlic's favorable effects on cholesterol.[3] Garlic preparations, including both fresh garlic and garlic oil, have also been found to stall or reverse atherosclerosis in rats, rabbits, and humans, reducing the size of lesions by nearly 50%.[4]

A German study published in 1990 was one of the largest human trials.[5] In this placebo-controlled randomized study, a total of 261 patients at 30 different medical centers were given either 800 mg of standardized garlic powder daily (containing 1.3% alliin) or placebo. At the start, average total cholesterol in the garlic group was 265 mg/dL and in the placebo group, 261. Average triglycerides was 223 and 216, respectively.

Over the course of 16 weeks, total cholesterol in the garlic-treated group fell 12% (compared to 3% in the placebo group) and triglyceride levels dropped 17% (compared to 2% in the placebo group). The greatest benefits occurred in patients with initial cholesterol levels of 250 to 300 mg/dL.

Another randomized, double-blind study conducted at Tulane University followed 42 healthy adults with a total cholesterol level of 220 mg/dL or higher.[6] The treated group received 300 mg 3 times daily of a garlic extract standardized to deliver 0.6% allicin. After 12 weeks, LDL cholesterol went down 11% in the treated group compared to 3% in the placebo group. Total cholesterol fell by 6% compared to 1%

**Garlic may lower total cholesterol by 6 to 12%, LDL cholesterol by 4 to 11%, and triglycerides by 17%.**

in the placebo group. HDL cholesterol, triglycerides, blood glucose, and blood pressure remained about the same.

Similarly positive results have been found in many other studies.[7] But not all studies have found solid benefits for garlic powder. One trial followed 115 individuals with total cholesterol concentrations of 231 to 328 mg/dL. Half of these received 900 mg daily of a garlic powder extract standardized to contain 1.3% allicin.[8] No significant difference was found between the treated and the placebo group.

Such varied results are perplexing, but they occur with approved conventional drugs as well. For example, some studies have found the antidepressant Prozac to be no more effective than placebo in the treatment of depression. On

## Carol's Story Continued: Trying Garlic

C arol, our typical patient from chapter 5, is considering giving garlic a trial run. She needs only a 10% drop in LDL cholesterol to reach her target goal of 160 mg/dL, and that appears to be within garlic's reach. She may not see her HDL cholesterol rise much, if at all, but it's already quite high. If garlic works, she will avoid dealing with the issue of flushing and other potential side effects associated with high-dose niacin therapy.

balance, the evidence for the effectiveness of garlic powder standardized to alliin content is fairly strong. There is also some evidence that aged garlic containing no alliin is effective.[9] However, garlic oil does not appear to work.[10]

## Other Cardiovascular Benefits of Garlic

Garlic may lower blood pressure. We'll discuss this further in chapter 13. The herb may also have anti-atherosclerotic effects independent of effects on cholesterol and high blood pressure.[11]

Like aspirin, garlic may thin the blood and make it less likely to clot, which could help prevent heart attacks and ischemic strokes. In a controlled (but not blinded) study of 432 individuals who had suffered a heart attack, those who took garlic oil had significantly fewer recurrent heart attacks (35%) and deaths (45%).[12] Remember that garlic oil does not appear to lower cholesterol. This may be a completely unrelated benefit.

And like vitamin E, garlic is an antioxidant.[13] This, too, may explain some of its apparent positive effects. Finally, garlic activates an enzyme called nitric oxide synthetase,[14] which may help arteries stay flexible.

# How Does Garlic Affect Cholesterol Levels?

Exactly how garlic works remains a mystery. Laboratory experiments on liver cells from chickens, monkeys, and rats have shown that allicin (and, to a lesser extent, ajoene) reduce the body's manufacture of cholesterol. These garlic components do this in the same way as statin drugs, by inhibiting the enzyme HMG-CoA reductase. They may also inhibit another enzyme (14 alpha-demethylase) involved in cholesterol production.[15] However, there is much we still don't know.

**Like vitamin E, garlic is an antioxidant.**

# Dosage

The general consensus is that one clove of raw garlic a day is an adequate dose for most conditions. The debate continues about the potency, efficacy, and proper dosage of various dried, aged, or deodorized garlic preparations. Cooked garlic may not be effective.

In most of the cholesterol studies, researchers used a dried form that supplies a daily dose of at least 10 mg of alliin, which can be converted into 4 to 5 mg of allicin (its "allicin potential"). From 1 to 4 months of therapy may be required to get the full effects.

However, not all manufacturers agree that allicin or alliin is even relevant to garlic's activity. Aged garlic preparations lack allicin and many other constituents of garlic. Still, there is some evidence that they can lower cholesterol, and they are very easy on the stomach.

Garlic is also sometimes sold preserved in oil. Such products contain no allicin or alliin, but do contain high levels of ajoene and dithiines and other breakdown products. As already mentioned, these have not proven effective in most studies.[16]

## Safety Issues

Garlic is on the Food and Drug Administration's GRAS (generally regarded as safe) list. Rats fed huge amounts of garlic extract (in proportion to their weights) for 6 months showed no significant toxicity[17] or genetic damage.[18]

An observational study followed almost 2,000 patients given 300 mg of garlic daily over a 16-week period.[19] The most frequent side effect was nausea. Rarer side effects included bloating, headache, sweating, dizziness, and allergic reactions.

Odor is the most common issue with garlic. Although so-called odorless products can help, they don't entirely eliminate the problem. One study suggests that therapeutic levels of odorless garlic produce an offensive garlic smell in half of participants, perhaps because of allicin formed in the digestive tract.[20] This can discourage people from continuing to take it, especially people whose jobs require them to interact with others.

Raw garlic taken in excessive doses can cause numerous symptoms, such as stomach upset, heartburn, nausea, vomiting, diarrhea, flatulence (gas), facial flushing, rapid pulse, and insomnia. Topical garlic can cause skin irritation, blistering, and even third-degree burns.

On largely theoretical grounds, garlic is not recommended for people with difficult-to-manage diabetes (garlic might lower blood sugar and thus interfere with blood sugar control); severe insomnia (garlic may worsen it); an abnormal skin condition called pemphigus (this disease can be activated by sulfur-containing compounds);

impending surgery or postsurgery (possible disturbance of blood clotting); organ transplants (possible activation of immune rejection); or acute rheumatoid arthritis (possible increase in autoimmunity).

Garlic in dietary doses is presumed to be safe in pregnancy and breastfeeding based on its extensive food use. However, the maximum safe dosage in these groups, as well as in those with severe liver or kidney disease, has not been established.

Garlic appears to thin the blood, so it could cause bleeding problems when combined with blood thinners such as aspirin or warfarin (Coumadin). For the same reason, you probably should not take large doses of garlic if you have bleeding problems or are scheduled for upcoming surgery, including dental surgery. There are at least theoretical concerns that garlic should not be combined with other natural blood thinners such as high-dose vitamin E and ginkgo.

Finally, if you use garlic to lower your blood cholesterol, you should see a medical professional and have your lipid levels followed. If garlic or other natural products fail to lower your cholesterol levels, don't simply experiment indefinitely. A 6-month trial should generally be sufficient. If your cholesterol levels don't improve, you should strongly consider using medications.

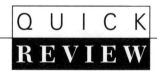

## QUICK REVIEW

- Garlic's use for many ailments is part of folklore.
- Allicin, one of its most important bioactive compounds, produces the characteristic odor associated with the herb.

- Garlic may lower cholesterol in the same way as statin drugs—by inhibiting a key enzyme required for its synthesis in the body—though the potential benefit of garlic is more modest.
- Garlic also appears to be an antioxidant and blood thinner.
- The studies of garlic have been mixed—not all have been positive: The results you get may depend on the form used. The general consensus is that one clove of raw garlic a day is an adequate dose for most conditions.
- From 1 to 4 months of therapy may be required to see the full effects.
- Garlic is generally regarded as safe.

# Other Natural Therapies for High Cholesterol

**M**any natural supplements are promoted as lowering cholesterol and thus helping to prevent heart disease. The evidence for most of them is not as convincing as for niacin, garlic, and vitamin E, but they warrant a brief look.

Two that do appear to be backed by good evidence are soy protein and sitostanol, and we will look at them first. The others in our discussion include red yeast rice, tocotrienols, essential fatty acids, glycosaminoglycans, pantethine, gugulipid, chromium, L-carnitine, calcium, and lecithin (phosphatidylcholine). A more complete discussion can be found in *The Natural Pharmacist Guide to Garlic and Cholesterol*.

## Soy Protein

Soy foods, once considered exotic, are now mainstream. Soy protein lowers cholesterol levels, and you should be seeing heart-healthy claims on the labels of foods containing it—such as soy milk, tofu, and vegetable burgers.[1] The Food and Drug Administration (FDA) says that the amino acids in soy protein, in combination with a healthful diet, can lower cholesterol and reduce your risk of heart disease.

**According to the FDA, you need to get about 25 g of soy protein daily to lower your cholesterol.**

You need to get about 25 g of soy protein daily to lower your cholesterol, according to the FDA. For labels to claim heart benefits, soy products must contain at least 6.25 g of soy—one-fourth the recommended daily level. Soy foods also appear to reduce your risk of cancer.[2]

You may even see soy burgers elbowing their way into traditional hamburger territory.

## Sitostanol

A new type of margarine containing sitostanol, a plant substance that substantially lowers cholesterol, may be available in the United States by the time you read this. In a Finnish study published in the *New England Journal of Medicine*, sitostanol lowered total cholesterol by 10% and LDL cholesterol by 14%.[3] Apparently, sitostanol has no affect on HDL cholesterol or triglycerides. It appears to work by preventing the absorption of dietary cholesterol from your digestive tract. Individuals in the study ate three pats of the margarine daily. Other plant-derived food products that push back cholesterol levels, such as salad dressings, are also expected to make it to your meal table.

# Red Yeast Rice

Red yeast rice is a traditional Chinese food and medicine made by fermenting the yeast *Monascus purpureus* on a bed of rice. This product is labeled as a dietary supplement for healthy men and postmenopausal women concerned about maintaining desirable cholesterol levels.

The formulation is standardized to contain 0.4% total HMG-CoA reductase inhibitors (the same compounds found in the prescription-only statin drugs; the first statin drug, lovastatin, was isolated from microorganisms). The product is said to contain 11 naturally occurring HMG-CoA reductase inhibitors; it may also contain flavonoids or other substances produced during fermentation.

Like statin drugs, red yeast rice appears to inhibit the enzyme called HMG-CoA reductase, which is the body's most important control point in its manufacture of cholesterol. Reduced production of cholesterol results in lower blood levels. However, HMG-CoA reductase inhibitors are present in very low amounts in red yeast rice, so it's possible that other factors may be at work.

## What Is the Scientific Evidence for Red Yeast Rice?

A double-blind placebo-controlled study followed 83 individuals given either 2,400 mg of red yeast rice daily or placebo for a period of 12 weeks.[4] The results showed an 18% drop in cholesterol in the treated group.

Most of the remaining research has been performed in China, and is not yet available in English. Reportedly, over 15 controlled studies have been performed, showing that blood cholesterol may be reduced from 11 to 32% with this product. However, without English versions of these studies, it is impossible to determine their validity. Additional U.S. research is underway at the present time.

## Dosage

The recommended dietary supplement dose is two capsules twice daily, morning and evening. To minimize gastrointestinal discomfort, take it with food and a beverage. Don't exceed four capsules in a 24-hour period.

## Safety Issues

Although there have been no serious adverse reactions reported in the studies of red yeast rice, some minor side effects have been reported. In the large study of 446 people, heartburn (1.8%), bloating (0.9%), and dizziness (0.3%) were all mentioned. Formal toxicity studies in rats and mice that were given doses up to 125 times over the normal human dose for 3 months showed no toxic effects, according to unpublished information on file with one of the manufacturers of red yeast rice.[5]

However, because red yeast contains ingredients similar to the statin drugs, there is a theoretical risk of the same side effects and risks that are seen with those drugs. These include elevated liver enzymes, damage to skeletal muscle, and increased risk of cancer. To be safe, if you have a history of liver disease or drink significant amounts of alcoholic beverages, you should avoid taking red yeast rice.

**Warning:** Red yeast rice should not be combined with niacin, erythromycin, cyclosporine or other immunosuppressive agents, other statin drugs, or the class of drugs called fibrates. Serious side effects, such as skeletal muscle damage and acute kidney failure have occurred when statin drugs were combined with these medications. Consult your physician if you experience muscle aches, unusual tiredness or weakness, or other adverse symptoms.

According to product labeling, the product should not be used if you're less than 21 years old; are pregnant or might become pregnant; are breastfeeding; have liver disease, a history of it, or risk factors for it; serious infections; a history of organ transplantation; a serious disease or physical disorder; or recent surgery.

## Tocotrienols

Tocotrienols are another recent over-the-counter dietary supplement said to lower cholesterol levels. The most popular product is a mixture of tocotrienols extracted from rice bran.

Tocotrienols are vitamin E–like compounds found naturally in foods such as rice bran and palm oil. Like vitamin E, tocotrienols are antioxidants, but they may also have other unique effects in preventing heart disease.

Tocotrienols appear to lower cholesterol levels similarly to statin drugs, garlic and red yeast rice—by inhibiting HMG-CoA reductase, resulting in reduced production of cholesterol by the liver and leading to lower blood levels of cholesterol. However, this isn't entirely proven. Tocotrienols may also inhibit blood-clotting.

### What Is the Scientific Evidence for Tocotrienols?

In test tube studies, tocotrienols have been found to inhibit HMG-CoA reductase activity and the manufacture of cholesterol. The type called gamma-tocotrienol showed a 30-fold greater activity compared to other tocotrienols.[6] But it's never easy to be certain that the results of laboratory studies like these apply to people. The concentration of tocotrienols achievable in a test tube are much higher than what you might take by mouth.

The few controlled trials on tocotrienols in humans that have been performed have produced varied findings. One researcher evaluated a proprietary mixture (tocotrienols containing vitamin E) in a controlled, double-blind study of 41 people with high cholesterol levels.[7] Total cholesterol fell by 16% and LDL cholesterol by 23% in the treatment group, compared to 7% and 11%, respectively, in the placebo group. (Why was there such a good effect in the placebo group? Perhaps because everyone in this study started to take better care of themselves.)

**Tocotrienols are vitamin E–like compounds found naturally in foods such as rice bran and palm oil.**

Another controlled trial found that the same branded tocotrienol mixture used in the above study may help protect against atherosclerosis, but, surprisingly, showed no benefit in lowering cholesterol.[8] Fifty people with cerebrovascular disease were followed over 18 months. Of the 25 treated individuals, plaque deposits appeared to improve in seven and to progress in two. None in the control group of 25 patients showed improvement, and 10 showed progression. But there was no change in cholesterol levels.

This directly contradicts the first study and leaves us somewhat in the dark as to whether tocotrienols actually work. Larger studies are needed to help sort out this tangle.

## Dosage

Not enough is known about tocotrienols to determine the best therapeutic dose. A dose frequently recommended is one to two 25-mg capsules daily. However, in one of the studies described above, a 220-mg tocotrienol mixture was used.

Some researchers suggest that vitamin E inhibits the effects of tocotrienols.

## Safety Issues

There are no known toxic effects at recommended doses, but safety studies have not been done. Pregnant or breastfeeding women and individuals with liver disease or other chronic disease should use this product only under medical supervision.

## Essential Fatty Acids

Fish contain omega-3 fatty acids, a form of polyunsaturated fat that may be protective against heart disease. Omega-3 fatty acids are "good fats" that are not made by the body and must be supplied by the diet or supplements. Interest in them began when it was found that natives of northern Canada who lived extensively on fish had few heart attacks despite a very high fat intake. Subsequent studies, however, have come to mixed conclusions.[9]

It appears that the omega-3 fatty acids produce little effect on total cholesterol levels, but significantly decrease serum triglycerides. They may slightly raise LDL cholesterol, but this effect is usually temporary.[10] Fish oil may also help prevent blood clots and lower blood pressure (we'll cover high blood pressure in chapters 11, 12, and 13).[11]

**Fish contain omega-3 fatty acids, a form of polyunsaturated fat that may be protective against heart disease.**

The bottom line is this: At the present time, it is not clear whether fish oil is beneficial for atherosclerosis and heart disease.[12]

One very odd result is that, like supplemental betacarotene, dietary fish (not fish oil) appears to be associated with a higher incidence of heart disease in smokers, according to an observational study.[13] The explanation for this is not clear. Due to the widespread publicity about the benefits of fish, it's possible that people with the worst heart health may have started eating fish, while most healthy people did not, muddling the study results. There are no end of complicating factors in observational studies!

Fish oil appears to be safe. Contrary to some reports, it does not seem to increase bleeding or affect blood sugar control in people with diabetes.[14]

Flax oil has been suggested as an alternative to fish oil.[15] However, there is no evidence that flax oil is effective, and it does not lower triglycerides. Flax oil, however, may stand on its own as a beneficial supplement for reducing the risk of cancer (See *The Natural Pharmacist Guide to Reducing Cancer Risk*).

# Other Herbs and Supplements for High Cholesterol

Several other natural supplements claimed to have beneficial effects on cholesterol merit brief mention, although there is no more than preliminary evidence that they might be helpful. Included in this group are glycosaminoglycans, pantethine, gugulipid, chromium, L-carnitine, calcium, and lecithin (phosphatidylcholine). More information about these substances may be found in *The Natural Pharmacist Guide to Garlic and Cholesterol.*

## Glycosaminoglycans

*Glycosaminoglycans* are substances found in high concentration in cartilage and the inside lining of arteries. Preliminary evidence suggests that supplementation with glycosaminoglycans may lower cholesterol and slow the progression of atherosclerosis.[16] It has been suggested that glycosaminoglycans may supply material for repairing blood vessel damage. A typical dose is 50 mg twice a day.

Glycosaminoglycans are regarded as safe because they occur widely in foods, but extensive safety studies have not been performed. Further research is needed to substantiate these preliminary findings.

## Pantethine

*Pantethine,* a special form of the vitamin pantothenic acid, may lower both triglycerides and cholesterol.[17] However, the evidence is still weak, and further research is necessary to evaluate the efficacy of this expensive supplement.

## Gugulipid

According to a few small studies, an extract of the Indian mukul myrrh tree known as *gugulipid* may reduce total cholesterol to a similar extent as garlic.[18] The proper dose of standardized guggul should supply 25 mg of guggulsterone 3 times a day. Side effects appear to be rare, but detailed safety studies have not been performed. More research is needed to substantiate the cholesterol-lowering effects of gugulipid.

## Chromium

The trace mineral *chromium* has shown primarily positive results on cholesterol levels, according to a 1993 review of 15 controlled studies of patients with impaired glucose tolerance (diabetes, for example).[19] Chromium was also found to decrease insulin resistance and thereby improve control of diabetes. Since diabetes is a risk factor for heart disease, in this way chromium may indirectly exert a beneficial

**The trace mineral *chromium* has shown primarily positive results on cholesterol levels.**

effect on heart disease. See *The Natural Pharmacist Guide to Diabetes* for detailed information on chromium.

## L-Carnitine

*L-carnitine,* an expensive amino acid supplement, has been promoted as a cholesterol-lowering agent, but there are few human studies evaluating its effects on cholesterol levels, and the current evidence is weak. One controlled study involved 160 patients of both sexes (ages 39 to 86 years) who had recently suffered a heart attack.[20] Eighty-one of these patients given L-carnitine (4 g daily) for 12 months showed clearly improved cholesterol levels. Several other cardiac benefits also emerged. These results are promising but very preliminary.

## Calcium

*Calcium* supplements may occasionally lower cholesterol, but more evidence is needed to confirm this benefit.[21] A typical nutritional dose is 500 to 1000 mg daily.

## Lecithin

The belief that *lecithin* has cholesterol-lowering activity was contradicted in a recent small, double-blind study of 23 men with high cholesterol levels. Researchers found that that lecithin treatment had no significant effects on blood levels of total cholesterol, triglycerides, HDL cholesterol, LDL cholesterol, or lipoprotein(a).[22] Lecithin is a major source of phosphatidylcholine, which the body breaks down into choline, a substance required for the proper metabolism of fats.

## Other Herbs

Many herbs may have an effect on heart disease through their actions on cholesterol or blood platelet stickiness. Most evidence comes from lab or animal studies, however, so it is difficult to draw firm conclusions. Herbs that may have some potential benefits include ginkgo, bilberry, ginger, green tea, feverfew, dong quai, grape seed, hawthorn, and turmeric. Natural substances that may help control blood pressure are discussed in chapter 13. See *The Natural Pharmacist: Your Complete Guide to Herbs* for more information.

Finally, general nutritional deficiencies can alter cholesterol levels, so it's probably a good idea to take a comprehensive multivitamin–mineral supplement.

# QUICK
# REVIEW

- Many natural supplements are claimed to lower cholesterol levels, but scientific evidence for many of them is limited.

- Soy protein appears to lower cholesterol levels. You need to get about 25 g daily to produce a significant effect.

- A new type of margarine containing the plant substance sitostanol may substantially lower LDL cholesterol, and similar plant-derived food products such as salad dressings are expected to become available.

- Red yeast rice appears to work similarly to the prescription-only cholesterol-lowering drugs called statins. U.S. studies are underway to further evaluate this traditional Chinese food. The recommended dietary supplement dose is two capsules twice daily, morning and evening. To minimize gastrointestinal discomfort, take it with food and a beverage. Don't exceed four capsules in a 24-hour period.

- Tocotrienols are vitamin E–like compounds found naturally in foods such as rice bran and palm oil. Not enough is known about tocotrienols to determine the best therapeutic dose. One to two 25-mg capsules daily is a typical recommendation.
- The evidence for essential fatty acids is somewhat disappointing, but they may lower triglycerides.
- Other herbs and supplements with possible cholesterol-lowering effects include glycosaminoglycans, pantethine, gugulipid, chromium, L-carnitine, calcium, and lecithin (phosphatidylcholine). Therapeutic doses for these agents have not been firmly established, and additional studies are needed to substantiate their benefits.

# Vitamin E and Other Antioxidants

**A**ntioxidant nutrients include vitamins E, C, A (includes beta-carotene), and the mineral selenium. They neutralize free radicals, highly unstable molecules that cause oxidative damage in the body. Other substances in foods also have antioxidant activity, and the body produces its own antioxidants. Free radicals are produced during normal body processes, from tissue injury, and also as a result of exposure to tobacco smoke, sunlight, x rays, and other environmental sources. Free radicals aren't entirely bad—the immune system uses them to destroy bacteria and other foreign invaders. Problems occur when the production of free radicals overwhelms the body's ability to contain them.

Extensive evidence suggests that damage by free radicals is in part responsible for heart disease, cancer, and other diseases associated with aging.

# Vitamin E

Vitamin E (tocopherol) is a fat-soluble antioxidant that plays a role in hemoglobin production, steroid metabolism, collagen formation, and in the metabolism of polyunsaturated fats (the type that help lower cholesterol).[1] Though there's no named deficiency disease that is the counterpart of scurvy (vitamin C deficiency) or rickets (vitamin D deficiency), a vitamin E deficiency results in central nervous system degeneration with symptoms such as impaired reflexes, movement, and vision.

**Antioxidants neutralize free radicals, highly unstable molecules that cause oxidative damage in the body.**

The major uses of vitamin E, however, do not consist of correcting a deficiency. Rather, they involve doses of vitamin E much higher than can reasonably be achieved through the diet. In these high amounts, vitamin E appears to offer considerable protection against heart disease, as well as other conditions. (For more information on vitamin E, see *The Natural Pharmacist: Your Complete Guide to Vitamins and Supplements.*)

## What Is the Scientific Evidence for Vitamin E?

There is more evidence for the effectiveness of vitamin E in heart disease than for any other antioxidant supplement, but much more research is needed. The CHAOS study, a randomized, double-blind, placebo-controlled intervention trial, followed 2,002 people with proven heart disease, for a period of almost 1.5 years.[2] One group took 800 IU of a vitamin E supplement daily, a second group took 400 IU

## What Is Daily Value?

**Y**ou have probably seen references on Nutritional Product labels to "DV." The new term *daily value* (DV) replaces the older term *recommended dietary allowance* (RDA). These values are designed to meet or exceed most people's requirements for that nutrient, and represent, in most cases, a wide margin of safety. Daily values are not minimal requirements—they contain an extra allowance for most groups of people.

daily, and the rest took placebo. The results were impressive: Those individuals given vitamin E had 77% fewer non-fatal heart attacks. This positive effect became apparent after taking the vitamin between 6 and 7 months. This is a significant benefit. Curiously, the vitamin E groups experienced slightly more heart-related deaths. It's not clear whether this was a significant finding or just a statistical aberration. More studies will be needed to clarify this point.

Observational studies strongly suggest that vitamin E helps prevent heart disease. A study that followed 39,910 U.S. male health professionals for 4 years found that vitamin E supplementation of 100 IU daily or more reduced the risk of heart disease by about 37%, compared to those not taking vitamin E.[3] Similarly good results have also been seen with women.[4]

One large study of 11,178 people aged 67 to 105 years found benefit from combining vitamins E and C. Those who were taking vitamin E supplements at the beginning of the study had a 34% lower risk of death from heart disease than those who were not. Vitamin C supplements alone did not seem to make a difference, but the combination of vitamins E and C boosted the risk reduction to 53%. Long-term use of vitamin E granted an even stronger risk reduction of 63%.[5] In this observational study, researchers made adjustments to rule out the influence of lifestyle and diet, and still arrived at substantially the same conclusion.

The apparent increased benefit provided by a combination of vitamins E and C suggests that these two antioxidants work as a team. Because vitamin E is fat-soluble and vitamin C is water-soluble, it makes sense that the two together might give broader protection against free radical damage. Indeed, research backs the idea that antioxidants in combination have an enhanced effect.[6]

**You need to take supplemental vitamin E to get the amounts generally associated with significant antioxidant activity.**

There have been some negative studies as well. Positive results were not seen in two other intervention trials of smokers given supplements of 50 IU of vitamin E daily.[7] It may be that vitamin E, especially at this relatively low dose, cannot overcome the powerful damaging effects of smoking.

Putting all the available evidence together, it is fair to say that vitamin E probably produces numerous heart benefits. More studies are needed to clarify its effects and determine the optimal dose.

## How Does Vitamin E Protect You Against Heart Disease?

Observational and animal studies suggest that vitamin E might help prevent oxidative damage to LDL cholesterol.[8] However, this is only a theory, and some evidence points against it.[9] LDL cholesterol, you may recall from chapter 1,

## Carol's Story Continued:
## Vitamin E Might Be a Good Idea

I t might be a good idea for Carol, our typical patient, to take vitamin E. She does not have heart disease, and vitamin E would appear to significantly lower her risk of getting it. Adding vitamin C might help even more by complementing the effects of vitamin E. To cover all the nutrient bases, she should also take a comprehensive multivitamin–mineral supplement.

plays a role in atherosclerotic plaque development. Oxidized LDL cholesterol may be even more harmful as part of this process.

Another explanation points out that, like aspirin, which is known to help prevent heart attacks, vitamin E makes blood platelets less sticky and thus less likely to clump together into dangerous blood clots.[10] But, again, we really don't know for sure.

## Dosage

The recommended daily value for vitamin E is 30 IU. However, the optimal dose of vitamin E for heart disease has not been determined. Studies suggest that at least 100 IU daily was required to reduce the risk of heart disease, and that 400 and 800 IU daily have a strong preventive effect against nonfatal heart attacks.[11]

Vitamin E may be absorbed better when you take it with food. You might also need more vitamin E if you eat large amounts of polyunsaturated fats.[12]

You may see vitamin E doses listed in either IU (international units) or milligrams (mg). Converting between IU and mg can be confusing, because vitamin E comes in several forms. For that reason, most sources just say that 1 mg

## What Is the Best Form of Vitamin E to Take?

**D**etermining the best form of vitamin E involves more than the natural versus synthetic question, but let's look at that issue first.

Taking 100 IU of synthetic vitamin E, for example, is supposed to be the same as taking 100 IU of natural vitamin E. However, a 1997 Japanese study reported that it took 400 IU of synthetic vitamin E to equal the blood levels obtained with just 150 IU of natural vitamin E.[13] The researchers concluded that natural vitamin E is almost three times more active in the body than the synthetic form, and that the natural form is therefore preferred for treating and preventing disease. Another study found similar results.[14]

How can you tell whether a product is synthetic or natural? Once you understand how to read the product label, it's easy. Vitamin E, like many other chemicals, comes in two mirror image forms—a right-handed (dextro or d) and a left-handed (levo or l) form. Synthetic vitamin E is made up of both forms, so it has "dl" in its name (e.g., dl-alpha-tocopherol). Natural vitamin E comes in only the "d" form (e.g., d-alpha-tocopherol). That's all there is to it.

of vitamin E is equivalent to 1 IU. That's certainly simple, but only correct for the synthetic form. Here's a guide:

- Synthetic vitamin E (dl-alpha-tocopherol) = 1.1 IU per mg.
- Natural vitamin E (in the form of d-alpha-tocopherol acetate) = 1.36 IU per mg.

But there's another important issue. Most vitamin E supplements contain only alpha-tocopherol, while foods contain several different tocopherols, including alpha-tocopherol and gamma-tocopherol. The gamma form appears to be important also.

A 1997 study found that the alpha and gamma forms of vitamin E may work best when taken together and that both may be necessary for optimal antioxidant activity. Additionally, taking the alpha form alone appeared to decrease blood levels of the gamma form.[15]

These studies suggest that the optimal vitamin E supplement would be the natural "d" form containing a mixture of tocopherols (including alpha and gamma).

However, all the scientific evidence we have for the effectiveness of vitamin E supplements comes from studies using alpha-tocopherol, so at this point we have no direct confirmation that mixed tocopherols are better. Some manufacturers may create confusion by calling the dl mixture (synthetic vitamin E) "mixed tocopherols," so read product labels carefully.

- Natural vitamin E (in the form of d-alpha-tocopherol) = 1.49 IU per mg.

Food sources, listed in order of higher to lower vitamin E content, include wheat germ oil, sunflower seeds and oil, almonds, hazelnuts, safflower oil, peanuts, cod-liver oil, peanut butter, corn oil, peanut oil, corn oil margarine, lobster, salmon, soybean oil, pecans. It's next to impossible to get the heart therapeutic doses of vitamin E from your (most people get 3 to 15 mg daily from the diet). Ex

for wheat germ oil (about 3( per tablespoon), other fc don't offer much. The nuts oils that do contain vitamin F also high in fats. You will n to take supplemental vita E to get the amounts gener associated with significant a oxidant activity.

> **One large study found benefit from combining vitamin E and C—the combination boosted the risk reduction to 53%.**

## Safety Issues

Vitamin E has an excellent sa record. Relatively large d( have been taken for exten periods without appar harm.[16] Most adults tole doses of up to 1,000 IU daily without adverse effects.[1

However, vitamin E's blood-thinning effect may incr the risk of hemorrhagic stroke (the type caused by a . tured blood vessel that bleeds into the brain).[18] On the o hand, vitamin E appears to reduce the risk of ischemic str the more common type caused by an obstructed blood sel to the brain, and this may outweigh the increased ris hemorrhagic stroke. In fact, a combination of vitamin E aspirin may in some cases help prevent ischemic stroke

**Warning:** Check with your physician if you take o blood thinners such as Coumadin (warfarin), aspi ibuprofen, or similar medications. Taking one of these d and vitamin E together may thin your blood too much increase the risk for abnormal bleeding. There are at I theoretical concerns that high-dose vitamin E should be combined with other natural blood thinners such as garlic and ginkgo.

# Vitamin C

Vitamin C (ascorbic acid) is a water-soluble antioxidant that acts as a preservative when added to foods. Deficiency symptoms include malaise, weakness, bleeding from small blood vessels, swollen gums, impaired wound healing, and bone changes. A profound deficiency of vitamin C is called scurvy.[20] Vitamin C has shown promise for many conditions, but the evidence is not yet strong that it is helpful in heart disease.

## What Is the Scientific Evidence for Vitamin C?

There have been about as many negative as positive studies regarding the benefits of vitamin C in heart disease.[21] The best evidence is that it may strengthen the beneficial effects of vitamin E and other antioxidant supplements.[22] As described earlier, since vitamin C is water-soluble and vitamin E is fat-soluble, both antioxidants together may cover a wider range of free radical damage.[23]

## Dosage

The adult recommended daily value for vitamin C is 60 mg.[24] An optimal dose to help prevent heart disease (probably in combination with vitamin E) is not known, but see the sidebar, What Is the Best Supplemental Dose of Vitamin C.

Food sources, listed in order of higher to lower vitamin C content, include acerola, guava, strawberries, papayas, orange juice, lemon juice, and grapefruit juice. Other foods in no particular order: broccoli, brussels sprouts, cantaloupe,

## What Is the Best Supplemental Dose of Vitamin C?

**V**ery large doses of vitamin C are often recommended some proponents, but a recent study suggests that 2 mg may be the optimal daily dose.[25] At a 200-mg single do bioavailability (the body's ability to use it) was complete. seems that about 200 mg a day saturates the body and most any higher dose is simply washed out in the urine. The researe ers concluded that the recommended daily value should increased to 200 mg (this much, they added, could be obtain from the diet), that safe doses of vitamin C are those less th 1,000 mg daily, and that vitamin C daily doses above 400 have no evident nutritional value. Although further research indicated, this finding does appear to mean that there is extra benefit in taking huge doses of vitamin C.

cauliflower, cranberry juice, honeydew melon, kiwi, man and tomato juice. The acerola fruit offers the biggest lo of vitamin C by far, with the fresh juice containing abc 1,300 mg of vitamin C per serving. A typical serving of t other foods in the ordered list provides about 40 to 242 of vitamin C each. You can easily get the recommend daily value of 60 mg from your diet, and it's not that di cult to get even 500 mg this way.

### Safety Issues

Vitamin C appears to be fairly nontoxic.[26] It has been ge erally believed that larger doses—over 1 g (1,000 n daily—can cause kidney stones, but recent studies have cast doubt on this assumption. In the large-scale Harvard Prospective Health Professional Follow-Up Study, those taking the most vitamin C (over 1,500 mg daily) had a lower risk of kidney stones than those taking the least amounts. Still, individuals with a history of kidney stones and those with kidney failure who have a defect in vitamin C or oxalate metabolism should restrict daily vitamin C intake to approximately 100 mg daily.[27]

Diarrhea may occur starting at 500 mg, but it usually goes away after a while. At about 4,000 mg, persistent diarrhea may occur. Cutting back on the dose should alleviate this side effect.

Because vitamin C is an acid (ascorbic acid), it can acidify the urine, which may diminish the effect of some medications. An acidic urine can also cause false results in diabetic urine tests. Finally, frequent chewing of chewable-type vitamin C tablets may cause some wearing down of your teeth due to the acid content. One tip is to crush the chewable tablets, dissolve them in water, and drink that. Or switch to the regular swallow tablets.

## Beta-Carotene

Beta-carotene is one of a family of substances called carotenes found in highest concentration in yellow/orange and dark green fruits and vegetables. The body can convert beta-carotene and other carotenes into vitamin A. Beta-carotene is a strong antioxidant, but it may not be as beneficial as other antioxidants when taken in supplement form. While numerous studies suggest that foods high in beta-carotene and other carotenes (fruits and vegetables) protect you against heart disease,[28] there is some evidence

## How to Get Your Beta-Carotene Without Taking a Supplement

With the jury still out on the value of beta-carotene supplementation, you might wish to forego supplements and get this nutrient from your diet. There are enough foods high in beta-carotene to make it feasible to get recommended antioxidant amounts from diet alone. The various forms of each of the foods below are listed in order from higher to lower beta-carotene content followed by the range in IU. Example: ½ cup mashed sweet potato contains approximately 28,000 IU of beta-carotene.

Sweet potato, ½ cup mashed, 1 baked, or 1 cup canned: 16,000 to 28,000 IU

Carrot, 1 raw or ½ cup boiled slices: 19,150 to 20,250

Spinach, ½ cup canned, frozen, or boiled: 7,300 to 9,400 IU (raw only 1,900 IU)

Mango, 1 medium: 8,100 IU

that beta-carotene in supplement form may actually increase the risk of heart disease, at least in smokers.

## What Is the Scientific Evidence for Beta-Carotene?

A double-blind intervention trial involving 29,133 Finnish male smokers found 11% more deaths from heart disease and 15 to 20% more strokes in those taking a beta-carotene supplement. Beta-carotene also increased the incidence of lung cancer. This is the same study that found little or no benefit on heart disease for vitamin E supplementation, but at least vitamin E didn't seem to be harmful.[29] The fact that beta-carotene actually worsened the outcome raised alarm balls throughout the medical community. As in many

Squash, butternut, ½ cup boiled: 7,150 IU

Squash, winter, ½ cup baked: 3,600 IU

Papaya, 1 medium: 6,100 IU

Cantaloupe, 1 cup: 5,200 IU

Turnip greens, ½ cup boiled or ½ cup raw: 2,150 to 4,000 IU

Mustard greens, ½ cup frozen or ½ cup boiled: 2,150 to 3,350 IU

You can get 50,000 IU (30 mg) of beta-carotene, for instance, from 1 cup of cooked sweet potatoes, 3 medium carrots, or 1 cup of cooked pumpkin. To get 25,000 IU (15 mg), eat ½ of a medium, cooked sweet potato, ½ cup cooked pumpkin, 1 ½ medium-sized carrots, 1 ½ cups of cooked spinach, or 2 medium-sized mangoes. Or mix and match as you like.

other studies, high levels of beta-carotene from food were found to be protective.

Another large double-blind study in smokers also found poor results with beta-carotene supplementation,[30] and beta-carotene supplements were found to increase the incidence of angina in smokers.[31] (You might ask why so many studies involved smokers. The reason is that it's easier to study the benefits of a preventive treatment in a group at high risk for the disease that treatment is thought to prevent.)

Why would foods high in beta-carotene protect against heart disease, while beta-carotene supplements do not? Several possibilities come to mind.

Beta-carotene may merely be a "marker" for a diet high in fruits and vegetables. In that case, it may be that other substances in these plant foods, such as carotenes, flavonoids, and sterols, confer the heart-protective effect. Or, beta-carotene may be protective only in the presence of other substances found in fruits and vegetables—the "teamwork" concept. It has also been suggested that taking beta-carotene supplements may promote deficiencies of other natural carotenes that may have protective benefits.[32] Finally, it is conceivable that beta-carotene may be harmful only for smokers, and for no one else.

Here's the bottom line: At our present state of knowledge, it appears to be wiser to eat yellow/orange and dark green vegetables than to take beta-carotene as a supplement.

## Dosage

A commonly recommended dose of beta-carotene is 25,000 IU daily.

Food sources, in order of higher to lower beta-carotene content, include sweet potato, carrots, spinach, mango, butternut and winter squash, papaya, cantaloupe, turnip greens, and mustard greens. Other foods, in no particular order, are broccoli, pumpkin, yellow corn, kale, apricot, and tomato.

## Safety Issues

High doses of vitamin A over long periods of time (25,000 IU or more) can be toxic. Although beta-carotene is turned into vitamin A, the body seems to be able to limit this conversion and avoid toxicity. The primary effect observed with very high beta-carotene doses (or drinking large amounts of carrot juice) is a dramatic yellowing of the skin. The condition disappears rapidly after stopping intake.[33]

Beta-carotene supplements may cause liver problems in heavy alcohol drinkers.

## Other Antioxidants

Besides vitamins E and C and beta-carotene, numerous other antioxidant vitamins, supplements, and herbs have been suggested as preventive treatments for atherosclerosis and heart disease. Selenium, procyanidolic oligomers (PCO) from grapeseed or pine bark, lipoic acid, turmeric, resveratrol (from red wine), soy isoflavones, $CoQ_{10}$, and garlic are commonly mentioned. While a number of interesting studies suggest these substances are beneficial, the results are highly preliminary.

Finally, fruits and vegetables as a group contain numerous antioxidants. There is very little doubt that higher amounts of these healthful foods in your diet help prevent heart disease, cancer, and other illnesses.

# QUICK
# REVIEW

- Antioxidants such as vitamin E and vitamin C can neutralize damaging molecules called free radicals. Free radicals may play a role in promoting heart disease as well as other chronic diseases such as cancer and diseases associated with aging.

- Foods high in antioxidants protect you against heart disease, but whether the benefits are due to the antioxidant vitamins, other naturally present antioxidants, or to some other substances present in foods is not known.

- Fairly solid evidence suggests that vitamin E in supplement form also helps protect you against heart disease. The recommended daily value for vitamin E is 30 IU. However, the optimal dose of vitamin E for heart disease may be higher. Studies suggest that at least 100 IU daily is required to reduce the risk of heart disease, and that 400 and 800 IU daily have a strong preventive effect against nonfatal heart attacks.

- The evidence is not as strong for vitamin C and other antioxidant supplements.
- A combination of antioxidants may work better than any one alone.

# Homocysteine and Heart Disease

**H**omocysteine has moved to center stage as a major independent risk factor for heart disease on a par with smoking and high cholesterol levels.[1] Medical researchers first became suspicious of homocysteine over 30 years ago, when they noticed that kids with a rare genetic disease died from heart disease at an early age. This particular genetic defect causes homocysteine blood levels to be very high. How might homocysteine be harmful? Laboratory research suggests that high levels may damage the inner artery lining and contribute to atherosclerotic plaque development, as well as promote blood clot formation.

Initially, the idea that moderately high homocysteine levels might be a heart disease risk factor for people in general did not receive a warm reception from the medical community, but recent research seems to have confirmed this view.

# What Is the Scientific Evidence Against Homocysteine?

A host of observational studies have suggested a link between too much homocysteine in the blood and an increased risk of heart disease and heart attack. One study found a two-fold increased risk of heart disease and another found a three-fold increased risk of heart attack.[2] A Norwegian study followed 587 patients with heart disease for almost 5 years.[3] The results showed that overall risk of death was 3.8% in those with the lowest levels of homocysteine, as compared to 24.7% in those with the highest levels.

**Homocysteine has moved to center stage as a major independent risk factor for heart disease on a par with smoking and high cholesterol levels.**

But homocysteine's role in heart disease may not be quite as straightforward as generally thought. In a recent study, published in the July 21, 1998, issue of *Circulation,* University of Minnesota researchers found *no* association between high homocysteine levels and risk of heart disease.[4] Instead, they found a connection between low levels of vitamin $B_6$ and increased heart disease risk. People with the highest vitamin $B_6$ levels were 28% less likely to get heart disease.

This finding brings up an interesting possibility. As we will discuss in chapter 10, vitamin $B_6$, folic acid, and vitamin $B_{12}$ are needed to keep homocysteine levels down. Deficiencies of these vitamins are associated with high blood levels of homocysteine. Could it be that high homocysteine levels are merely a marker for low levels of vitamin $B_6$? Could homocysteine be an innocent bystander rather than a key villain?

It's too early to say, but the latest findings have at least temporarily jarred out of focus our once sharp picture of homocysteine's role in heart disease. Randomized clinical trials are now underway to refocus the picture.

Whether the connection to heart disease turns out to be high homocysteine or low vitamin $B_6$, taking supplemental $B_6$ helps in either case. Using B vitamins to lower elevated homocysteine levels is the subject of chapter 10.

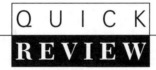

- It's generally believed that homocysteine contributes to atherosclerotic plaque development, and that high blood levels of this naturally occurring amino acid are a major risk factor for heart disease.

  A recent study casts doubt on this idea and suggests instead that low vitamin $B_6$ levels may be a risk factor.

  Research is underway to clarify this important issue.

CHAPTER
**TEN**

# Using B Vitamins to Control High Homocysteine

**A**s we learned in chapter 9, deficiencies of the B vitamins folic acid, $B_6$, and $B_{12}$ can lead to elevated homocysteine levels. Numerous studies have found that supplementation with these vitamins can lower elevated homocysteine levels. Additionally, some studies have found that B-vitamin supplementation may also diminish your risk of heart disease.

## What Is the Scientific Evidence for B Vitamins?

The Framingham Heart Study, one of the classic gold mines of heart-related health information, found an important link: If your intake of $B_6$, folic acid, or $B_{12}$ is low, your homocysteine levels are likely to be high. Furthermore, about two-thirds of the people studied were not getting enough $B_6$ or folic acid in their diet. ($B_{12}$ deficiency is much less common.)

Other studies have found that supplementation with folic acid and vitamin $B_6$, alone or in combination with each other, lowers homocysteine levels.[1] Vitamin $B_{12}$ supplementation also appears to help. One clinical trial found that B-vitamin supplementation in men with moderately high homocysteine levels reduced these levels by more than half.[2] In this particular study, the doses used were well above nutritional doses: folic acid (1,000 mcg), vitamin $B_6$ (10 mg), and vitamin $B_{12}$ (50 mcg).

However, as mentioned in chapter 9, we don't know for sure that high homocysteine levels cause heart disease, so these findings can't be taken as proof that supplemental B vitamins will protect against heart disease.

We do know that low blood levels of folic acid and vitamin $B_6$ have been linked to an increased risk of heart disease.[3] But, as mentioned several times in this book, just because people with heart disease have low levels of folic acid and $B_6$ doesn't mean that taking extra folic acid and $B_6$ will help. It is always possible that heart disease causes the vitamin deficiency, rather than the reverse.

**Numerous studies have found that supplementation with folic acid, vitamins $B_6$, and $B_{12}$ can lower elevated homocysteine levels.**

What we really need are some intervention trials where people are given $B_6$ and folic acid or placebo, and the rate of heart disease is evaluated. Such clinical trials are currently underway. At the present time, the best evidence we have comes from an observation study, the Nurses' Health Study. (That large study of 121,700 female nurses ages 30 to 55 began in 1976. Like the Framingham study, it has provided a motherlode of valuable health information.)

The study, published in the February 4, 1998, issue of the *Journal of the American Medical Association*, examined data on 80,000 of the women in the Nurses' Health Study who had no history of heart disease. Researchers looked at their intake of folic acid and vitamin $B_6$ to check for a possible connection between that and the development of heart disease.[4]

Vitamin intake from both diet and multivitamin supplementation was considered. It was found that women with the highest folic acid intake had half the risk of heart disease compared to those with the lowest intake, and that each 100 mcg/day increase in intake lowered the risk by 5.8%. Positive results were also seen with vitamin $B_6$ intake—in this case, each 2 mg/day increase in intake lowered the risk by 17%. The routine use of multiple vitamins in supplement form reduced the risk of heart disease by 24%.

**The routine use of multiple vitamins in supplement form reduced the risk of heart disease by 24%.**

Additionally, women who got at least 400 mcg/day of folic acid and 3 mg/day of vitamin $B_6$ were significantly less likely to suffer heart attacks compared to those who got much lower amounts. Researchers concluded that higher intake of folic acid, either alone or in combination with vitamin $B_6$, significantly reduced the risk of heart disease and heart attack in women.

These results are impressive and are an important addition to our store of information, but we must consider the observational nature of this study. The data on vitamin intake used by the researchers came from questionnaires on health and lifestyle filled out by the nurses over the course of several years. As with all such studies, there is no way to know whether some unidentified factor may have played a role in the results.

The positive finding for vitamin $B_6$ takes on even more meaning in light of the study discussed in chapter 9. That study suggested that vitamin $B_6$ levels may be more important than homocysteine levels as a risk factor for heart disease. Clearly, there is more work to be done to accurately nail down the interplay between levels of homocysteine, B vitamins, and heart disease.

Despite the fact that the evidence is not yet set in stone, it certainly makes sense to get enough $B_6$, $B_{12}$, and folic acid in your diet anyway. A multivitamin supplement might typically provide 400 mcg of folic acid, 2 mg of vitamin $B_6$, and 6 mcg of vitamin $B_{12}$. This may be all the protection most people need.

**Researchers concluded that higher intake of folic acid significantly reduced the risk of heart disease and heart attack in women.**

## Folic Acid

Folic acid (Folacin) is one of the water-soluble B vitamins. It functions in concert with vitamin $B_{12}$ in many body processes, such as amino acid metabolism, DNA and protein synthesis, cell division, and development of the nervous system and fetus. Research suggests that higher intake of folic acid, either alone or in combination with vitamin $B_6$, significantly reduces the risk of heart disease and heart attack in women.

## David's Story

**R**ecently, my friend David, 52, casually asked me after a tennis game what I thought about vitamin supplementation. David has been trying to control his slightly high blood pressure with diet and exercise. The other day, his doctor suggested that he take a multivitamin supplement "just to be on the safe side."

From what he told me, his cholesterol was slightly high, but he had no history or symptoms of heart disease. He takes medicine only when he can't avoid it. "I don't believe in vitamin supplements," he said. "What do I need those extra vitamins for?"

I knew David had two risk factors for heart disease—high blood pressure and his gender/age (male, over age 45). I discussed his heart disease risks and told him that I believed in

---

Folic acid deficiency is the most common vitamin deficiency worldwide, and deficiency during pregnancy is associated with birth defects. Deficiency symptoms include sore mouth, diarrhea, and central nervous system symptoms, such as irritability and poor memory.[5]

## Dosage

The adult recommended daily value for folic acid is 400 mcg.[6] However, only about 10% of people in the United States get 400 mcg daily.[7] To help you get more dietary folic acid, the government now requires that flour, breads, and breakfast cereals be fortified with the vitamin. That will generally add about an extra 100 mcg a day, but most people will still not get 400 mcg a day by diet alone. Most multivitamin supplements contain 400 mcg.

prevention where possible. I was pretty sure he had not had his homocysteine levels measured. But our discussion about homocysteine, B vitamins, and heart disease risk caught his interest.

I told him that many people don't get high enough levels of B vitamins from their diet and that taking a comprehensive multivitamin supplement would be a painless way to get the B vitamins "just in case your levels might be high." I also mentioned other benefits of good vitamin coverage.

Last week, he told me that he and his wife were both taking the multivitamin–mineral supplement I recommended. I decided to wait a while before suggesting extra vitamins E and C (see chapter 8)—I didn't want to hit him with too much at once.

The optimal dose of folic acid for lowering homocysteine levels has not been clearly determined. A 1997 study found that three widely varying doses of folic acid supplementation reduced homoscysteine levels by the same amount—30%. The daily doses were 400 mcg, 1 mg (1,000 mcg), and 5 mg (5,000 mcg) taken over a 3-month period.[8]

One recommended treatment regimen is to start with 400 mcg/day and recheck homocysteine levels in 4 to 6 weeks. Another suggests that high-risk patients with moderately high homocysteine levels (over 12 umol/L) start with 1,200 mcg/day, with 400 mcg supplied by a standard multivitamin supplement and 800 mcg provided by a folic acid supplement. If homocysteine levels are normal after 8 weeks, cut back to taking only the multivitamin supplement (400 mcg folic acid). If homocysteine levels have not responded, gradually increase the folic acid dose up to 5 mg/day.[9] If you have chronic kidney failure, you will need a much higher dose.[10]

In addition to folic acid from the diet, women of childbearing age should take an extra 400 mcg daily in supplement form to prevent neural tube birth defects such as spina bifida in their babies.

Food sources, in order of higher to lower folic acid content, include brewer's yeast, blackeyed peas, soy flour, wheat germ, beef liver, soybeans, wheat bran, kidney beans, lima beans, asparagus, lentils, walnuts, fresh spinach, peanut butter, broccoli, whole-wheat cereal, brussels sprouts, almonds, oatmeal, cabbage, avocado, green beans, corn, pecans, blackberries, and oranges.

## Safety Issues

Folic acid presents little risk of toxicity. It is water soluble and is rapidly eliminated from the body. Up to 15 mg has been given daily without toxic effects, but high doses (5 to 10 mg) may cause annoying gastrointestinal symptoms, such as nausea and appetite loss.[11] A 1996 review concluded you could take doses up to 5 mg daily without being too concerned about harmful effects.[12]

Several drugs may increase your need for folic acid. The anticonvulsant phenytoin (Dilantin) and related drugs may inhibit folic acid absorption.[13]

**Warning:** Do not take more than 800 mcg of folic acid daily without a doctor's evaluation. It may mask the signs of vitamin $B_{12}$ deficiency while irreversible nerve damage progresses.

# Vitamin $B_6$ (Pyridoxine)

Vitamin $B_6$ is a water-soluble B vitamin that contributes to numerous enzymes. Among other functions, it helps the body metabolize amino acids.

## Dosage

The recommended daily value for vitamin $B_6$ is 2 mg for most adult men and 1.6 mg for most adult women.[14] A typical multivitamin supplement contains 2 mg.

In the studies described earlier, a 3 mg daily dose was found to be heart-protective. For those with heart disease, 4 mg daily has been suggested.

Foods rich in vitamin $B_6$ include meats, cereals, lentils, nuts, and some fruits and vegetables, including bananas, avocados, and potatoes. The average diet provides slightly less than the recommended daily value.

## Safety Issues

In excessive doses, vitamin $B_6$ can be toxic, producing symptoms of nerve disease. Such symptoms have appeared in doses as low as 150 mg, although they usually do not appear until 300 mg a day or more.

Also, vitamin $B_6$ can work against the therapeutic effect of levodopa by preventing its active form from reaching the brain. If you take levodopa (for Parkinson's disease, for example), you should avoid vitamin $B_6$ supplements. This is probably not a problem with Sinemet (levodopa combined with carbidopa), but you should check with your doctor to be safe.

# Vitamin $B_{12}$ (Cyanocobalamin)

Vitamin $B_{12}$ is a water-soluble B vitamin that plays a role in fat, protein, and carbohydrate metabolism. Deficiency is less common than with the other B vitamins discussed in this chapter, because vitamin $B_{12}$ can be stored for a long period of time. However, among people of retirement age and older, there are conflicting reports on the prevalence of deficiency with estimates ranging from 5 to 42%.[15]

## Dosage

The adult recommended daily value for vitamin $B_{12}$ is 6 mcg. Most multivitamin products contain 6 mcg.

People with reduced levels of stomach acid (such as those taking ulcer medication) may not absorb $B_{12}$ well from foods. The acid is needed to separate $B_{12}$ from protein. Taking $B_{12}$ in supplement form does not present this problem.

A daily dose of 6 mcg is suggested for a heart-protective benefit. If you already have heart disease, 8 mcg daily has been recommended.

Vitamin $B_{12}$ is found naturally in foods of animal origin such as meats, oysters, and clams.

## Safety Issues

Vitamin $B_{12}$ appears to be essentially nontoxic, even in very high doses.

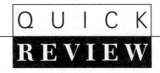

QUICK
REVIEW

- B vitamins, especially folic acid and vitamin $B_6$, have been found to lower elevated homocysteine levels.
- The evidence is highly suggestive that such supplementation may also reduce your risk of heart disease, and clinical trials to confirm this are underway.

  The recommended protective doses are 400 to 1,200 mcg (folic acid), 3 to 4 mg (vitamin $B_6$), and 6 to 8 mcg (vitamin $B_{12}$). Higher doses have been used in some studies.

  An over-the-counter multivitamin supplement may supply sufficient amounts of these vitamins for most people.

# High Blood Pressure and Heart Disease

T he term hypertension may conjure up a picture of "tension" or "nervousness." (One student of mine, thinking the term referred to some type of emotional disorder, chose hypertension as the topic for an assigned paper.) In fact, hypertension is the technical name for high blood pressure. The disease is not caused by stress or tension, but may in some cases be aggravated by them. It's important to realize you can have high blood pressure and still feel calm and well.

You might give little thought to your blood pressure. Yet one in every four Americans has high blood pressure, and many of them are not even aware they have it. That oversight can be dangerous: High blood pressure is known as the "silent killer" because telltale symptoms may not be apparent. Damage occurs behind the scenes—the longer you let it go, the more damage done. That's why doctors check your blood pressure each time you come in for a visit. If you don't go to the doctor often, you should try to get your blood pressure checked at least twice a year. If you already know you have high blood pressure, it's a good idea to check it even more frequently, perhaps by monitoring it yourself with a home blood pressure device.

## What Is High Blood Pressure?

Ordinarily, the heart beats steadily at about 60 to 70 times a minute. With each beat, it pumps a spurt of blood out to the body. The pressure created against blood vessel walls

**One in every four Americans has high blood pressure, and many are not even aware of it.**

as the heart pumps and rests is your blood pressure. The higher pressure generated at the peak of the pumping action is called systolic pressure. The lower pressure between pumps is called diastolic pressure. In a blood pressure reading, systolic pressure is the first number listed, followed by the diastolic number—for example, 135/87.

Blood pressure varies with physical activity and sometimes with strong emotion and stress. Usually, artery walls expand and contract to maintain a steady flow of blood to body tissues during both rest and exercise. When you stand up, the body makes various adjustments so the blood supply to the brain is not drained by gravity.

You may find it surprising to know that most people (95%) with high blood pressure have no known cause for the disease. This is called *primary hypertension* or essential hypertension. The other 5% have *secondary hypertension,* for which a cause can be identified. Often, this second type

## Who Gets High Blood Pressure?

**P**redicting who might get high blood pressure is not always possible, but individuals with certain risk factors may be more likely to develop it.

- High blood pressure affects African Americans more often than whites and Mexican Americans.
- In African Americans, it tends to occur earlier in life and be more severe.
- Blood pressure tends to rise with age. Hypertension is more common in men up to about age 60, when the tables turn and it becomes more common in women.
- This disease is also inherited to some degree. If your parents or other relatives have had elevated blood pressure, the chances are greater that you will too.

is easier to treat, since removing the cause usually alleviates the high blood pressure. Although we don't know what causes primary hypertension, it appears to result from unidentified alterations in kidney function and blood vessel tension.

Blood pressure tends to vary from day to day. The issue really is not whether your blood pressure is high at any one time, but whether it remains high chronically. The definition of stage 1 hypertension is blood pressure above 140/90 on three separate occasions. About a third of people who register high blood pressure on a single reading will not have an elevated reading the next time. A single extremely high reading may require immediate care, but this is uncommon.

## Jack's Story: "White Coat" Hypertension

J ack had just been to the doctor and was getting a prescription filled for his cold symptoms. The nurse at the doctor's office had taken his blood pressure, and she had mentioned something about needing to keep an eye on it because it was at the high end of normal. She had written the numbers down for him. While he waited at the pharmacy, he decided to get a blood pressure reading at the blood pressure machine near the waiting area.

This reading turned out to be several points lower than what it had been at the doctor's. Jack was pleased, but he was puzzled by the apparent discrepancy. He mentioned this to the pharmacist, who said it might be a case of "white coat hypertension." That's what it's called, the pharmacist explained, when you have an increase in blood pressure during a visit to the doctor. "It's not uncommon," he said.

# How Does High Blood Pressure Increase Heart Disease Risk?

Like elevated cholesterol, high blood pressure accelerates atherosclerosis. You may recall that the initial step in the development of atherosclerotic plaque—the process underlying heart disease—is damage to the inner artery wall. High cholesterol levels in the blood can damage the arteries. Such damage can also be caused by the prolonged mechanical stress of high-pressure blood flow against artery walls. Imagine a garden hose with the nozzle closed and the water left

What does this mean for you? For one thing, if you measure your blood pressure at home and find it to be lower than it was at the doctor's office, you can't necessarily accept the lower reading at face value. When the standards for normal blood pressure were set, they were based on readings at the doctor's office. Many people have higher blood pressure there than they do at home. Also, if your blood pressure rises under the stress of a doctor's visit, it's also probably rising in traffic, at work, and during family conflicts. So if your blood pressure is high at the doctor's office but not at home, you probably still need to do something about it.

Here's something else so basic it may be overlooked: Avoid tobacco or caffeine a couple of hours before taking a blood pressure reading, since these can affect blood pressure. Also, blood pressure taken within two hours after a meal, especially in an older individual, may be artificially low.

on full-bore; once or twice doesn't matter, but if you do this all the time the hose will rapidly deteriorate under the strain.

The eventual result of atherosclerosis, as we've discussed in early chapters, may be a stroke, angina, or a full-blown heart attack. Artery walls in the kidney and retina (of the eye) may also suffer damage. Even mild high blood pressure, left untreated, can injure the kidneys. This has been found to be the source of damage in about a fourth of patients undergoing kidney dialysis.

Additionally, chronic high blood pressure makes the heart muscle enlarge so it can pump harder against this pressure. Over time, this may cause the heart to weaken and be unable to pump as much blood as your body needs. When that happens, blood begins to back up into the lungs and legs, a condition known as congestive heart failure. Chronic high blood pressure may lead to declining mental function in the elderly by promoting numerous small strokes. For all these reasons, managing high blood pressure is extremely important. In chapters 12 and 13 we will discuss how to bring your blood pressure down.

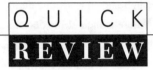

## QUICK REVIEW

- Hypertension or high blood pressure is a major risk factor for heart disease.
- High blood pressure is called the "silent killer" because telltale symptoms may not be apparent.
- The disease damages artery walls and contributes to the development of atherosclerotic plaque, the process underlying heart disease.
- It can also damage the kidneys, eyes, and other parts of the body.
- Additionally, it can lead to heart failure and declining mental function.

# Conventional Therapies for High Blood Pressure

L ifestyle changes and drug therapy—the conventional ways to tame high blood pressure—have yielded dramatic benefits, including a 53% decline in deaths from heart disease and an almost 60% drop in deaths from stroke over the last several decades.[1] Before going further, let's take a brief look at how blood pressure is classified to see where you stand.

## How Is Blood Pressure Classified?

The latest guidelines for the treatment of high blood pressure were published in 1997. They are part of the sixth report of the Joint National Committee on Prevention, Detection, Evaluation, and Treatment of High Blood Pressure (called JNC VI). The report classifies blood pressure into several stages for adults age 18 and older. (See table 5, Blood Pressure Classifications.)

Within each of the three stages of hypertension, you fall into one of three risk groups according to the number of risks you have, such as high cholesterol, diabetes, or smoking. Your risk group determines whether your initial therapy should be lifestyle changes or drug therapy. For example, if you have stage 1 high blood pressure and are otherwise at low risk, like David in chapter 10, you would be treated with lifestyle modifications alone for 6 to 12 months. Lifestyle modifications include dietary changes, weight loss, quitting smoking, and regular exercise. If that did not bring your pressure under control, drug therapy would be considered.

Traditionally, the cutoff number for high blood pressure was considered to be 140/90. Numbers below these were considered normal. However, recently this level has been lowered. Now the *optimal* blood pressure with respect to heart disease risk is considered to be below 120/80 (as shown in table 5). In the past, medical professionals believed that lowering diastolic pressure (the lower number) too much might increase certain risks. However, the current view is that, barring extremes, the lower your pressure, the better off you are.

**Blood pressure shoots up with each cigarette smoked.**

Also traditionally, doctors focused on diastolic pressure much more than systolic pressure. Today, however, doctors believe systolic pressure may also be very important. A high systolic pressure, even with a normal diastolic pressure, increases the risk of stroke, especially in older people.

When the two numbers in a blood pressure reading fall into different hypertension stages, the higher stage is used. For example, a reading of 162/92 would put you in stage 2 hypertension (your diastolic pressure is stage 1, but your systolic pressure is stage 2). A reading of 174/120 puts you

## Table 5. Blood Pressure Classifications (JNC VI)

| Category | Blood Pressure (mm Hg) | |
| --- | --- | --- |
| | Systolic | Diastolic |
| Optimal | <120 | <80 |
| Normal | <130 | <85 |
| High-Normal | 130–139 | 85–89 |
| Stage 1 hypertension | 140–159 | 90–99 |
| Stage 2 hypertension | 160–179 | 100–109 |
| Stage 3 hypertension | ≥180 | ≥110 |

Note: < (less than), ≥ (greater than or equal to)

into stage 3 (your systolic pressure is stage 2, but your diastolic pressure is stage 3).

## Lifestyle Modifications: Your First Step

As with heart disease in general, lifestyle modifications should be your foundation for controlling high blood pressure. This includes eating a healthful diet, getting regular exercise, losing weight, stopping smoking, and limiting alcohol intake (see the sidebar, Lifestyle Modifications to Prevent and Manage Hypertension). These changes can lower blood pressure and reduce the need for drug therapy.

You should always try lifestyle modifications before drug therapy, unless your blood pressure is extremely high or accompanying diseases make immediate action necessary. Many people can manage high blood pressure (or prevent it from occurring) with lifestyle changes alone. If you do require drug therapy, you may need fewer drugs and lower doses if you make these changes.[2]

## Stop Smoking

Smoking is seriously damaging for several reasons. It's an independent major risk factor for heart disease. The nicotine in cigarettes is a stimulant and blood pressure shoots up with each cigarette smoked. Blood pressure medications may not lower heart disease risk in smokers as much as in nonsmokers.[3] Quit smoking if at all possible. Check with a local hospital about available smoking cessation resources. A program might include nicotine replacement therapy and/or the prescription drug bupropion.

## Limit Your Alcohol Intake

Drinking too much alcohol has several drawbacks: It can raise blood pressure, interfere with the effects of blood pressure medications, and increase the risk of stroke. (See the sidebar, Lifestyle Modifications to Prevent and Manage Hypertension for recommended limits.) On the other hand, moderate alcohol intake may lower blood pressure, and these limits are in line with the evidence that two drinks a day for men and one for women may lower the risk of heart disease in middle-aged adults.

**Obesity goes hand in hand with increased blood pressure. A weight loss of as little as 10 pounds (4.5 kg) can nudge your blood pressure down.**

## Reduce Your Body Weight

Obesity goes hand in hand with increased blood pressure. Specifically, obesity refers to a body mass index (BMI) of 27 or more. (See the discussion of body weight in chapter 4 for more on how to calculate your BMI.) A weight loss of as little as 10

## Lifestyle Modifications to Prevent and Manage Hypertension

- Stop smoking.
- Limit your alcohol intake to no more than 1 ounce ethanol daily for men and 0.5 ounce daily for women and persons of lighter weight. (1 ounce of ethanol is equivalent to 24 ounces of beer, 10 ounces of wine, or 2 ounces of 100-proof whiskey.)
- Reduce your body weight if you are overweight.
- Increase your aerobic physical activity to 30 to 45 minutes most days of the week.
- Cut your sodium intake to 2,400 mg daily or less (1 level teaspoon of salt contains about this much).
- Maintain an adequate intake of dietary potassium.
- Maintain an adequate intake of dietary calcium and magnesium.
- Reduce your intake of dietary saturated fat and cholesterol for overall heart health.

pounds (4.5 kg) can nudge your blood pressure down. Weight loss also makes blood pressure medication work better.

## Increase Your Physical Activity

Increasing your aerobic physical activity brings a host of benefits. It helps in both prevention and treatment of high blood pressure. Besides lowering blood pressure and helping you lose weight, it reduces your risk of heart disease and death from all causes. All it takes is moderate exercise, such as a brisk walk for 30 to 45 minutes most days of the week. (See the discussion of exercise in chapter 4 for more details.)

## Eat a Healthful Diet

"Dietary Approaches to Stop Hypertension (DASH)," a recent study, showed that improvements in diet can substantially lower your blood pressure whether it is high or not (generally, lowering blood pressure even when it is not high is beneficial).[4] The recommended diet is similar to that of the AHA and to recommendations in the Food Guide Pyramid. (See the topics Diet and Lifestyle: Your Best Defense Against High Cholesterol and The Food Guide Pyramid: Your Map to Healthful Eating in chapter 4.) The DASH diet is rich in fruits, vegetables, and lowfat dairy foods, and low in saturated fat and total fat. It's also high in fiber and the minerals potassium, calcium, and magnesium.

## Cut Back on Dietary Salt (Sodium)

Dietary salt (sodium chloride) refers to the kind found in a salt shaker at the meal table. For years, salt was thought to be bad for blood pressure across the board. Now it seems that only about half of people with high blood pressure are "sensitive" to salt. African Americans appear to be especially salt-sensitive, as do the elderly and those with diabetes.[5]

**Inadequate dietary potassium is linked to increased blood pressure.**

Just cutting back moderately on salt can reduce medication needs and provide other benefits. The improved food label makes it easy to choose low-sodium foods. (See The Nutrition Facts Food Label in chapter 4.)

## Get Adequate Dietary Potassium

Too little potassium in the diet is linked to increased blood pressure.[6] Boosting dietary intake may help prevent high

## What About Coffee?

**C**affeine (found in coffee and colas) can increase blood pressure considerably, but the body appears to adapt with moderate regular intake so that pressure goes down again. No precautions appear necessary except in individuals with other reasons to limit caffeine consumption.[7] However, don't overdo it. For instance, regularly drinking 4 or 5 cups in the morning may be potentially harmful.

blood pressure and improve control in those who have the disease. We'll look at potassium in detail in chapter 13.

## Drug Therapy for High Blood Pressure

Controlling blood pressure with drug therapy reduces the risk of heart disease, heart attack, stroke, heart failure, kidney disease, and deaths from all causes.[8] Unfortunately, getting people to stay on their medication is a major problem.

High blood pressure may have no apparent symptoms until a heart attack or stroke hits. So it's easy to think, *Why do I need pills when I don't feel sick?* Also, the medication itself often has side effects, so you may actually feel better when you don't take it. Typically, people may wind up stopping their pills and not returning to see the doctor. The unfortunate result: Their blood pressure climbs back up and continues its steady assault unnoticed.

The side effects you might experience early in therapy may clear up after a while. If they don't, your doctor may have to experiment a bit to find the best medications in the right doses for your particular needs. There are so many types of blood pressure medications available that it's usually possible to find one that does not cause troublesome

## Can Religious Belief Ease Blood Pressure?

A recent observational study of 112 women who were at least 35 years old and were of a variety of Judeo-Christian faiths found a direct benefit of religious beliefs on blood pressure.[9] Information on general health behaviors such as physical activity, smoking, diet, and alcohol consumption was measured by questionnaire.

Improvements in both systolic and diastolic blood pressure suggested that religious feelings may lower blood pressure directly, such as by improving ability to cope with stress. Generally, diastolic pressure was more affected than systolic, and factors called "intrinsic religiosity" and "religious coping" were found to be most influential. Additionally, "religious experiences" may exert a greater beneficial effect on diastolic blood pressure in older age groups (50 to 80 years). Researchers said the results supported a direct relationship between religious feeling and blood pressure, rather than an indirect effect through modification of other health behaviors.

side effects. Some good news is that drug therapy may not have to last forever. In some cases, it's possible to reduce doses (called step-down therapy) and even stop drug therapy if you can get your blood pressure under control with lifestyle modifications.

## Types of Drugs Used for High Blood Pressure

Several types of drugs are used to treat high blood pressure. They include diuretics, ACE inhibitors, angiotensin II receptor-blockers, beta-blockers, alpha-blockers, calcium channel-blockers, and direct vasodilators.

## Diuretics

Diuretics used to be the most popular treatment for high blood pressure, and evidence suggests that they can reduce the incidence of heart disease and deaths. Initially, they help rid the body of excess sodium and fluid, but we aren't sure exactly how the reduction in blood pressure they bring is maintained. The long-term effect appears to be a decrease in blood vessel resistance, which lightens the workload on the heart. Diuretics are especially effective if your blood pressure is sensitive to salt intake. They also enhance the effect of most other high blood pressure medications.

In low doses, diuretics have minimal side effects. Higher doses may temporarily increase your blood sugar and cholesterol levels. They may also wash too much potassium out of your body, resulting in hypokalemia (low potassium levels), a potentially dangerous situation. To offset this, extra potassium may be prescribed in the form of a salt substitute containing potassium or a prescription-only potassium supplement. Or the doctor may prescribe a type of diuretic that does not deplete potassium. Other possible side effects include sexual dysfunction, gastrointestinal upset, gout, diarrhea, dizziness or lightheadedness, and appetite loss.

Diuretics should not be used routinely during pregnancy and should be avoided during the first month of breastfeeding.

## ACE Inhibitors

Presently, a different class of drug, the ACE inhibitors (angiotensin-converting enzyme inhibitors), have taken over the "preferred" position. They have been shown to reduce your risk of heart attack, stroke, and death if you have high blood pressure.[10] They may also benefit you if you've had a heart attack.

ACE inhibitors interfere with the body's production of an enzyme that causes your kidneys to retain salt and fluid and your arteries to constrict. Their most common side effect is a dry cough. Other possible side effects include postural hypotension (see the discussion of alpha-blockers, below), skin rash, impaired taste, hyperkalemia (high potassium levels), headache, sluggishness, nausea, and breathing difficulties. In clinical practice, many doctors have found these agents to cause fewer side effects than other drugs for high blood pressure.

ACE inhibitors should not be used during pregnancy, especially the second or third trimester. The drug should be stopped as soon as pregnancy is detected. Use cautiously in breastfeeding.

### Angiotensin II Receptor-Blockers

Angiotensin II receptor-blockers, the newest high blood pressure medications, produce beneficial effects similar to ACE inhibitors, but don't give you their most common side effect, a dry cough.

The same pregnancy and breastfeeding precautions associated with ACE inhibitors apply.

### Beta-Blockers

Beta-blockers have also been found to reduce heart disease and deaths. They make your heart beat more slowly and with less force by blocking nerve impulses that produce the opposite effects. Possible side effects include sluggishness, depression, sexual dysfunction, dizziness or lightheadedness, drowsiness, and insomnia. Certain beta-blockers may worsen congestive heart failure or asthma.

Beta-blockers should be used cautiously in pregnancy and breastfeeding.

### Alpha-Blockers

Alpha-blockers block nerve impulses that tell blood vessels to constrict, allowing your arteries to relax and open wider. Some of these drugs may cause a condition called postural hypotension—a sudden drop in blood pressure causing dizziness or faintness when you arise after sitting or lying down. Other possible side effects include drowsiness, depression, headache, constipation, dry mouth, and swelling of feet or ankles.

These drugs should be used cautiously during pregnancy and breastfeeding.

### Calcium Antagonists (Calcium Channel–Blockers)

Calcium channel-blockers have been found to protect individuals who have had a heart attack. They cause your blood vessels to relax and open wider, as well as make the heart beat more slowly and with less force. They do this by preventing the movement of calcium into heart cells and blood vessels. Muscles, including those in the heart and blood vessels, need calcium to contract.

A few years ago, controversy over the safety of one of the immediate-acting calcium antagonists was widely publicized. It appears now that this story was much overblown. The important point is that no serious adverse effects have been shown for the long-acting agents approved for the treatment of high blood pressure.

Possible side effects include constipation, sluggishness, dizziness or lightheadedness, flushing and feeling of warmth, diarrhea, headache, and nausea.

These agents should be avoided in pregnancy unless clearly needed, and should be used cautiously during breastfeeding.

### Direct Vasodilators

Direct vasodilators act directly on your blood vessel walls to relax them and allow them to open wider. Common side effects may include dizziness, headache, irregular heart rhythms, nausea, vomiting, and fluid retention.

They should be avoided in pregnancy unless clearly needed. Potential effects in breastfeeding are not known.

## Drug Therapy Considerations

There are many opinions and guidelines concerning what type of drug to start with in individuals with high blood pressure. Generally, doctors start with a low dose of one drug and work upward as needed. Older people should be started on about half the dose used in younger people. It may take a few months of drug therapy to find a combination of the best dose and fewest side effects. A switch to a different medication may be called for; or you may need to take a combination of drugs to get proper control of your blood pressure.

The ideal agent is one that has a 24-hour action. That means you need to take it only once a day. This is a big convenience and helps you stay on drug therapy. Even more important, it provides smooth control of blood pressure and protects you in the critical early morning hours. Blood pressure is highest in the morning after awakening. It's essential that your blood pressure therapy be dosed to cover this vulnerable time.

Though the JNC VI guideline does not recommend mineral supplements or other natural supplements for managing blood pressure, several recent studies suggest they may help. That's the subject of the next chapter.

# QUICK
# REVIEW

- Controlling high blood pressure helps protect you from heart disease and many other damaging conditions.

    Lifestyle modifications are usually your first step in managing high blood pressure.

    These include dietary changes, weight loss, smoking cessation, and regular exercise.

- If those don't work, drug therapy may be needed.

    One problem with drug therapy is getting people to stay on their medication.

    Medication may cause unpleasant side effects until the right drug and dose are determined.

    In some cases, it's possible to reduce doses and even get off drug therapy if a good blood pressure can be maintained with lifestyle modifications.

# Nutrients and Herbs That Lower High Blood Pressure

**A** growing body of evidence suggests that supplementing dietary needs with certain nutrients and herbs may help control high blood pressure. These supplements are useful for moderate high blood pressure, 160/110 or less. For more severe blood pressure elevation, drug treatment is usually necessary. However, some of these treatments (such as the minerals) may be usefully combined with medication. Among the natural agents that show evidence for lowering blood pressure are the minerals potassium, magnesium, and calcium, as well as coenzyme $Q_{10}$, garlic, fish oil, flaxseed oil, and hawthorn.

Keep in mind that 5% of cases of high blood pressure—the type called secondary hypertension, as discussed in chapter 11—have an identifiable cause that must be directly treated. So make sure to see a physician to rule this out before self-treating.

# Minerals

Animal and epidemiological studies suggest that various dietary minerals influence blood pressure. Sodium (common table salt) tends to increase blood pressure, and decreasing intake lowers it. Potassium, magnesium, and calcium may lower blood pressure.[1] In clinical trials of mineral supplementation for high blood pressure, the evidence is strongest for potassium; results for magnesium and calcium have been inconsistent.

## Potassium

A diet deficient in potassium is linked to increased blood pressure.[2] Getting more from the diet may help prevent high blood pressure and improve control if you have the disease.

In several small trials, the effect of potassium appears to be definite but modest: an average decline of 3.11 mm in systolic blood pressure and 1.97 mm in diastolic blood pressure.[3] The effect was greatest in those who also consumed a lot of sodium, which suggests that potassium can balance out sodium's tendency to raise blood pressure in some people. People with severe hypertension experienced the greatest pressure-lowering effect, and this effect was more pronounced the longer they took potassium. Taking extra potassium also improved blood pressure control in individuals with low potassium levels caused by diuretic drugs. Reviewers concluded that increasing potassium intake should be included in the nondrug management of patients with uncomplicated hypertension.

## Magnesium

Numerous animal studies have suggested that magnesium deficiency leads to hypertension.[4] People with long-term hypertension appear to have at least a 15% deficit in magnesium levels.

However, results of studies on the effect of supplemental magnesium on blood pressure have varied. It may depend on the form of magnesium used—studies showing benefit used magnesium oxide, while other studies showing no effect used a different form of magnesium. Other factors may also play a role.[5] Overall, the benefit of magnesium appears to be slight.

## Calcium

More than 80 experimental studies have reported lowered blood pressure after increasing dietary calcium.[6] A major review of human studies using supplemental calcium found a very small benefit.[7] Calcium supplementation was associated with a small reduction in systolic pressure (1.27 mm) and an even smaller reduction in diastolic pressure (0.24 mm). The authors pointed out that these results do not rule out a better benefit of calcium in some individuals.

**Reviewers concluded that increasing potassium intake should be included in the nondrug management of patients with uncomplicated hypertension.**

## How Can You Get the Minerals You Need?

The blood pressure reductions associated with mineral supplementation appear to be modest at best. These nutritional supplements are probably best viewed as an adjunct to other treatments. Even so, it makes sense to get the recommended daily value of these minerals. The best source for them as well as other nutrients for overall good health is your diet. In a healthful diet, minerals and other components may all work together in beneficial ways. If you are deficient in any of these minerals or cannot consume an adequate diet, supplementation may be called for.

The recommended daily values for potassium and magnesium are 4 g (4,000 mg) and 400 mg, respectively. You can easily get this much from the diet. For example, one banana has 400 mg of potassium and an ounce of all-bran cereal contains 106 mg of magnesium.

For calcium, the recommended daily value is 1,000 mg for adults and 1,200 mg for those over age 50. Many people don't get this much in their diets (nonfat milk, for example, contains about 300 mg of calcium per 8 ounce serving). In this case, a supplement is advisable.

- High dietary sources of calcium include dairy foods, fish and meat substitutes, vegetables, and grains.
- Good sources of potassium include fresh fruits and vegetables; unprocessed meats and poultry; fish; and milk, cheese, and yogurt.
- The richest dietary sources of magnesium are green leafy vegetables; tofu (a soy product); beans and legumes; breads, cereals, and other whole grains; and nuts and seeds.

## Coenzyme $Q_{10}$ (Ubiquinone)

In Japan and other countries, coenzyme $Q_{10}$ ($CoQ_{10}$) is an approved treatment for several cardiovascular conditions. Considerable evidence suggests that it may be useful in treating congestive heart failure as well as other heart conditions. For these purposes, it is often combined with conventional medications. (See *The Natural Pharmacist: Your Complete Guide to Vitamins and Supplements* for more information.) $CoQ_{10}$ has also been proposed as a treatment for high blood pressure.

$CoQ_{10}$ was first identified as an orange-colored substance present in heart muscle cells of cows. Eventually, it was found to exist in many human organs, including the

**CoQ₁₀ is made by the body and also is ingested from foods such as meats, fish, and soybean oil.**

heart, kidney, liver, and pancreas. It is made by the body and also is ingested from foods such as meats, fish, and soybean oil. It turns out that $CoQ_{10}$ helps cells turn food into energy, so it's found almost everywhere in your body. For that reason, it's also called ubiquinone, a name derived from the word ubiquitous (existing everywhere). Since the body can synthesize $CoQ_{10}$ from other substances, it is not classified as an essential nutrient.

$CoQ_{10}$ has antioxidant effects, working like vitamin E to neutralize free radicals and thus prevent the cell damage caused by them.[8] It may also help recycle used-up vitamin E.[9]

## What Is the Scientific Evidence for Coenzyme Q₁₀ in High Blood Pressure?

It's been suggested that $CoQ_{10}$ may lower your blood pressure by reducing the resistance of blood vessels to the flow of blood. However, there is little actual research evidence. Most of the studies performed lacked a control group.

One placebo-controlled trial of $CoQ_{10}$ has been performed, but it was very small, involving only 18 hypertensive patients.[10] They received either 100 mg of $CoQ_{10}$ daily or a placebo for 10 weeks. In the $CoQ_{10}$ patients, systolic and diastolic pressures fell by 10.6 mm and 7.7 mm, respectively. The placebo group showed no changes in blood pressure. These are promising results that need to be confirmed in larger studies.

In a small non-placebo trial, 26 people with hypertension received a 50-mg dose of $CoQ_{10}$ twice a day for 10 weeks. The results showed about a 10% improvement in blood pressure.[11] Another non-placebo trial of 109 patients treated with $CoQ_{10}$ also showed a significant improvement in blood pressure over a period of 1 to 6 months.[12] However, because many studies have shown that even placebo pills can lower blood pressure (as well as

**$CoQ_{10}$ has antioxidant effects, working like vitamin E to neutralize free radicals and thus prevent the cell damage caused by them.**

inspire participants to make lifestyle improvements), we really need double-blind placebo-controlled trials to know whether $CoQ_{10}$ really works.

As promising as $CoQ_{10}$ supplementation might seem, the research evidence for its blood pressure-lowering effects must be regarded as preliminary only.

## Dosage

The dose of $CoQ_{10}$ for treating hypertension, congestive heart failure, and other conditions has been 30 to 150 mg daily or more, divided into two or three doses at the higher levels. Duration of therapy has lasted as long as 6 years.

$CoQ_{10}$ is fat-soluble and is better absorbed when taken in oil-based soft-gel form rather than in a dry form such as tablets and capsules.[13]

## Safety Issues

No serious side effects have been reported with $CoQ_{10}$ therapy. Infrequent side effects have included gastrointestinal discomfort, nausea, diarrhea, and appetite loss. But since it's been studied only in small trials, we can't be certain it's entirely safe.

HMG-CoA reductase inhibitors—such as the lipid-lowering statin drugs discussed in chapter 4—may lower body levels of $CoQ_{10}$ and lead to a deficiency in it.[14] Taking supplemental $CoQ_{10}$ may be a good idea if you are taking one of these medications.

Drug interaction studies have not been done.

Maximum safe doses in young children, pregnant or breastfeeding women, or those with severe liver or kidney disease has not been established.

**Warning:** $CoQ_{10}$ treatment for heart conditions should be supervised by a physician.

# Garlic

Numerous studies have suggested that garlic lowers blood pressure modestly.[15] Taken together, the seven best studies suggest that garlic powder may lower systolic pressure about 7.7 mm and diastolic pressure about 5 mm more than placebo.

In one 12-week study, 47 people with blood pressures averaging 171/101 were treated with either 600 mg of garlic powder daily or placebo.[16] The results showed a statistically significant drop of 11% in systolic pressure and

13% in diastolic pressure compared to only 5% and 4%, respectively, in the placebo group.

The review authors concluded that garlic appears to be mildly effective for high blood pressure, but that better research is needed before garlic can be recommended as a useful treatment for this condition.

A recent study suggested that garlic's blood pressure–lowering effect may escalate over time. In this 16-week open trial, 80 patients with high blood pressure were given either a standardized garlic preparation or garlic oil.[17] In those taking the standardized preparation, systolic pressure dropped by 10% after 4 weeks and by 19% after 16 weeks. Diastolic pressure showed similar progressive decreases. The amount of standardized garlic preparation given was 600 mg 3 times daily (an unusually high dose) standardized to 1.3% alliin.

There was no benefit in the garlic oil group. However, because the average blood pressure in this group was significantly lower at the start, comparisons cannot be fairly drawn.

For more on the herb garlic, including dosage and safety issues, see chapter 6 and *The Natural Pharmacist Guide to Garlic and Cholesterol.*

## Fish Oil

A 1993 review of clinical trials found that fish oil supplements (a source of omega-3 fatty acids) appear to modestly lower blood pressure in individuals with untreated hypertension.[18] Omega-3 fatty acids are essential fatty acids that are not made by the body and must be supplied by the diet or supplements. The doses of omega-3 fatty acids used were high—generally more than 3 g daily. The effect was greater in those with higher blood pressure.

However, there are many flaws in this research. The authors concluded that further studies are necessary before omega-3 fatty acids can be recommended for treating high blood pressure.

## Flaxseed Oil

Flaxseed, a high-fiber grain cultivated since ancient Egyptian times, may be a good alternative to fish oil for some uses. Fish oils are rich in the omega-3 fatty acid eicosapentaenoic acid (EPA). While flaxseed oil does not contain EPA, it does contain the omega-3 fatty acid alpha-linolenic acid, which can be converted to EPA in the body.

Dietary linolenic acid in general appears to be associated with lower blood pressure, according to a study that analyzed the fatty tissue content of 399 people.[19] Researchers found that each 1% increase in dietary linolenic acid was associated with a 5 mm decrease in systolic, diastolic, and average blood pressure. Keep in mind that this was an indirect study and may not translate to a direct effect of treatment.

One tablespoon of flaxseed oil taken daily is typically recommended to meet the body's essential fatty acid needs.

## Hawthorn

Hawthorn, a shrub tree widely used as a hedge plant in Europe, may lower blood pressure slightly. The herb is a member of the rose family, but its white flowers emit an unpleasant odor altogether different from the dreamy fragrance of its kin.

It may work by causing blood vessels to open wider and other mechanisms.[20] Some studies, though, have not shown this effect. More evidence exists for its use in congestive heart failure. (The other herbal treatment for congestive heart failure, foxglove, became the conventional heart drug, digitalis.) Hawthorn is also used for angina.

In general, clinical studies have shown that hawthorn does not affect heart rate or blood pressure at rest but does help hold them down during exercise.[21]

Because of its high content of procyanidins, hawthorn has also been proposed for the same uses as grape seed, such as prevention of atherosclerosis. (See chapter 7.)

The herb is also widely recommended by herbalists as a treatment for the minor, typically harmless irregular heart rhythms called "heart palpitations," though there is no direct scientific basis for this use.

The standard dose of hawthorn is 100 to 300 mg 3 times daily of an extract standardized to contain about 2 to 3% flavonoids or 18 to 20% procyanidins. Hawthorn appears to require 4 to 8 weeks to be effective. Single doses produce little effect.[22]

**In general, clinical studies have shown that hawthorn does not affect heart rate or blood pressure at rest but does help hold them down during exercise.**

Germany's Commission E lists no known risks or contraindications with hawthorn.[23]

Side effects include mild gastrointestinal distress and allergic reactions. There are no known drug interactions, but such studies have not been performed. Because hawthorn clearly has effects on the heart, the possibility of interactions with other cardiovascular drugs should not be ignored.

Safety in young children, pregnant or breastfeed
women, or individuals with severe kidney or liver dise
has not been established.

For more information on hawthorn, see *The Natu
Pharmacist: Your Complete Guide to Herbs.*

**Warning:** Hawthorn has potent effects on the heart
its use should be supervised by a doctor.

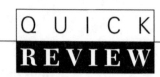

- Lifestyle and dietary modifications may help you avoid
ting high blood pressure.

    If you have high blood pressure, such changes may en
    you to treat it with fewer drugs and lower doses.

    In some cases, you might even be able to avoid drug the
    altogether.

- Supplementing your dietary needs with certain nutrients
herbs may add extra benefits.

    Among the natural agents that show some evidence for
    ering blood pressure are the minerals potassium, magnes
    and calcium.

    Other promising substances include coenzyme $Q_{10}$, ga
    fish oil, flaxseed oil, and hawthorn.

- The recommended daily dosages are:

    potassium (4,000 mg)

    magnesium (400 mg)

calcium (1,000 mg for adults and 1,200 mg for those over age 50)

coenzyme $Q_{10}$ (30 to 150 mg or more)

garlic (1 clove fresh garlic; dose differs with other forms)

fish oil (over 3 g has been used, but lower doses may produce similar effects)

flaxseed oil (1 tablespoon)

hawthorn (300 to 900 mg)

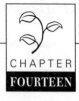

CHAPTER
**FOURTEEN**

# Putting It All Together

**F**or your easy reference, this chapter contains a brief summary of key information contained in this book. Please refer to earlier chapters for more comprehensive information, including a detailed discussion of safety issues.

Heart disease is the number one disease killer in the United States. Its dire consequences include angina, heart attack, congestive heart failure, and stroke.

Your first line of defense against the disease consists of dietary and lifestyle modifications to control its major risk factors: high cholesterol levels, high blood pressure, high homocysteine levels, smoking, physical inactivity, being overweight, and diabetes. Doing this can stall heart disease in its tracks and perhaps even coax its retreat.

Certain nutrient and herbal supplements may complement dietary and lifestyle modifications, further protecting you against heart disease. If your physician says it's okay to spend some time exploring natural therapies, you can try these. For safety information, see the topics for the various natural agents.

Drug treatment should be considered when nondrug therapies don't work well enough.

# Natural Treatments for High Cholesterol

High cholesterol, especially high LDL cholesterol, is a major risk factor for heart disease. Here are some natural approaches to controlling your cholesterol.

## Diet

Diet is the cornerstone of your cholesterol-lowering efforts. Eat a lowfat, low-cholesterol, high-fiber diet. You can do this by emphasizing fruits and vegetables, whole grains, lean meats, and monounsaturated fats, such as olive oil or canola oil.

## Exercise

Physical inactivity is a welcome mat for heart disease. Regular, moderate physical activity builds your overall cardiovascular fitness and helps control not only high cholesterol, but also high blood pressure, obesity, and diabetes. All it may take is about 30 minutes at least 3 times a week. A key to sticking with exercise is to find the type you enjoy—it can be weight training, aerobics, walking, swimming, or sports activities—anything that gets you up and going!

## Niacin

Niacin (nicotinic acid) in high doses lowers LDL cholesterol and triglycerides and raises HDL cholesterol (the good kind). There are ways to minimize its pesky side effects, such as the skin reaction called flushing. Begin with a lower dose, such as 50 to 100 mg 3 times daily, taken with or just after meals. Increase the dose 100 to 250 mg every 7 to 14 days. The goal dose is generally 500 to 1,000 mg 3 times daily.

Liver toxicity, a more serious potential problem, is associated more often with the slow-release form of niacin. There are many complicating factors, so you should discuss with your physician which form would be better for you (regular or slow-release niacin). Make sure you have regular blood tests to monitor liver function.

## Garlic

Garlic is the best-documented herbal treatment for high cholesterol. In most of the studies that evaluated the cholesterol-lowering effects of garlic, researchers used a powdered form that supplies a daily dose of at least 10 mg of alliin, which may be listed as a total allicin potential of 4 to 5 mg. You may need to take it 1 to 4 months to get the full effects. Garlic is also sometimes sold preserved in oil. Such products contain no allicin or alliin but high levels of ajoene and dithiines and other breakdown products. These have not proven effective in most studies.

## Other Natural Treatments for High Cholesterol

Numerous other supplements may also be effective for lowering cholesterol.

### Soy Protein

Soy protein, found in foods such as soy milk, tofu, and vegetable burgers, contains amino acids that lower cholesterol. The FDA plans to allow labels on certain products to claim they may reduce your heart disease risk.

### Sitostanol

The plant substance sitostanol appears to substantially lower LDL cholesterol and is the ingredient in a new type of margarine. Similar plant-derived food products such as salad dressings are also expected to become available.

### Red Yeast Rice

Red yeast rice is a traditional Chinese food and medicine. Studies done in China suggest a substantial cholesterol-lowering effect, but these findings are preliminary, and more studies are needed.

### Tocotrienols

Tocotrienols, vitamin E–like compounds, possess antioxidant effects and may lower cholesterol, as well as exert other unique effects. As with red yeast rice, larger studies are needed to evaluate the potential benefits.

### Essential Fatty Acids

The evidence regarding a cholesterol-lowering effect for essential fatty acids, such as omega-3 fatty acids found in fish oil and flaxseed oil, is somewhat disappointing, but they may lower triglycerides.

### Other Herbs and Supplements

Other herbs and supplements with possible cholesterol-lowering effects include glycosaminoglycans, pantethine, gugulipid, chromium, L-carnitine, calcium, and lecithin (phosphatidylcholine). Therapeutic doses for these agents have not been firmly established.

## Antioxidants and Heart Disease

Antioxidants such as vitamin E, vitamin C, and beta-carotene help neutralize damaging molecules called free radicals, which may play a role in heart disease.

## Vitamin E

Supplemental vitamin E appears to protect you against heart disease and heart attacks, as well as other serious heart problems. It works as both an antioxidant and blood thinner. The recommended daily value for vitamin E is 30 IU. The optimal dose of vitamin E for heart disease has not been determined, but studies show that at least 100 IU daily was required to reduce the risk of heart disease and that 400 and 800 IU daily had a strong preventive effect against non-fatal heart attacks. Supplemental vitamin E may be absorbed better when taken with food.

## Vitamin C

Supplemental vitamin C may find its most important role against heart disease as a secondary player. It may enhance your overall protection when combined with vitamin E and other antioxidants. The recommended daily value for vitamin C is 60 mg, but much higher doses are typically taken.

## Beta-Carotene

Although it is an antioxidant, there is no evidence that beta-carotene in supplement form is helpful, and it may even increase the risk of heart disease. Beta-carotene and other carotenes present in fruits and vegetables, however, do seem to be beneficial.

# Natural Treatments for High Homocysteine

It's generally believed that homocysteine contributes to atherosclerotic plaque development. High levels of this amino acid, found naturally in the blood, are thought to be a major risk factor for heart disease—on a par with high cholesterol levels and smoking.

## Folic Acid, Vitamin B$_6$, and Vitamin B$_{12}$

These B vitamins help break down homocysteine and eliminate it from the body. If you have high levels of homocysteine, taking supplemental doses of these vitamins may help lower it.

The recommended therapeutic doses are 400 to 1,200 mcg folic acid; 3 to 4 mg vitamin B$_6$; and 6 to 8 mcg vitamin

$B_{12}$. Higher doses have been used in some studies. A multivitamin supplement might typically provide 400 mcg of folic acid, 2 mg of vitamin $B_6$, and 6 mcg of vitamin $B_{12}$. This may be all the protection you need. Before taking larger doses, you should have your risk assessed and homocysteine levels checked, and remain under a doctor's care for periodic monitoring.

# Natural Treatments for High Blood Pressure

High blood pressure (hypertension) is another major risk factor for heart disease. The prolonged mechanical stress of high-pressure blood flow against your artery walls damages them. The injured area is a fertile bed for atherosclerotic plaque development and subsequent heart disease. High blood pressure also damages many other areas in your body.

## Lifestyle Modification

Appropriate lifestyle and dietary modifications help you in many ways. You may be able to avoid getting high blood pressure in the first place. If you have high blood pressure, you may be able to treat it with fewer drugs and lower doses. In some cases, you might even be able to avoid drug therapy altogether.

Lifestyle modification includes getting regular exercise, losing weight, stopping smoking, and limiting alcohol intake. The recommended diet is similar to that for heart disease itself: Emphasize foods low in saturated fat and total fat and high in fiber and the minerals potassium, calcium, and magnesium—such as fruits, vegetables, and lowfat dairy foods. For exercise recommendations, see Natural Treatments for High Cholesterol.

## Natural Agents

Many natural agents may modestly lower your blood pressure.

## Minerals

Of the minerals, evidence for a blood pressure–lowering effect is strongest for **potassium**, while results for *magnesium* and *calcium* have been inconsistent. It makes good sense to limit your intake of dietary **sodium**, which can elevate blood pressure. Magnesium may also be beneficial in congestive heart failure.

The recommended daily values for potassium and magnesium are 4 g (4,000 mg) and 400 mg, respectively. You can easily get this much from your diet. For example, one banana has 400 mg of potassium, and 1 ounce of all-bran cereal contains 106 mg of magnesium.

For calcium, the recommended daily value is 1,000 mg for adults and 1,200 mg for those over age 50. Many people don't get this much in their diets (nonfat milk, for example, contains about 300 mg of calcium per 8-ounce serving). In this case, a supplement is advisable.

## Coenzyme $Q_{10}$

Coenzyme $Q_{10}$ (ubiquinone), a natural body substance, helps cells turn food into energy. It's been suggested that $CoQ_{10}$ may lower your blood pressure by reducing the resistance of blood vessels to the flow of blood. However, the best evidence for $CoQ_{10}$ is in the treatment of congestive heart failure. It may also help in cardiomyopathy (an enlarged or weakened heart).

The dose for treating cardiac-related conditions has been 30 to 150 mg daily or more, given in two or three divided doses at the higher levels.

$CoQ_{10}$ is fat-soluble and is better absorbed when taken in oil-based soft-gel form rather than in a dry form, such as tablets and capsules. $CoQ_{10}$ is often added to a conventional drug regimen to boost the effects. However, it is not wise to self-treat these serious conditions without medical supervision.

# General Cautions That Apply to All Natural Agents

- The maximum safe dosage in young children, pregnant or breastfeeding women, or those with severe liver or kidney disease has not been established.
- Treatment for all cardiovascular diseases should be supervised by a physician.

## Garlic

Garlic, in addition to its cholesterol-lowering effects, may modestly lower blood pressure.

## Omega-3 Fatty Acids

*Fish oil supplements* are a source of omega-3 fatty acids, and may lower blood pressure slightly. High doses—over 3 g daily—were used in the studies, but lower doses may also work.

*Flaxseed oil* is also a source. One tablespoon of flaxseed oil taken daily is typically recommended to meet the body's essential fatty acid needs.

## Hawthorn

The herb hawthorn has potent effects on the heart. It may lower blood pressure slightly, but finds its most important use in congestive heart failure. It's also used for angina. The standard dose of hawthorn is 100 to 300 mg 3 times daily of an extract standardized to contain about 2 to 3% flavonoids or 18 to 20% procyanidins. Single doses produce little effect. Hawthorn may require 4 to 8 weeks to be effective. Again, medical supervision is necessary for optimum effects.

# Notes

## Chapter One

1. Strong JP, et al. Early lesions of atherosclerosis in childhood and youth: natural history and risk factors. *J. Am. Coll. Nutr.* 11: 51S–54S, 1992; Strong JP. The natural history of atherosclerosis in childhood. *Ann. N.Y. Acad. Sci.* 623: 9–15, 1991.

2. Davidson M, et al. Confirmed previous infection with Chlamydia pneumoniae (TWAR) and its presence in early coronary atherosclerosis. *Circulation* 98 (7): 628–633, Aug 18, 1998.

3. Beck JD, et al. Periodontitis: a risk factor for coronary heart disease? *Ann Periodontol* 3 (1): 127–141, Jul 1998.

4. Overmyer RH. Treating atherosclerotic disease: current strategies. *Formulary* 33 (Suppl. 1): S3, 1998.

5. Source: American Heart Association.

6. Kannel WB, Belanger AJ. Epidemiology of heart failure. *Am Heart J.* 121: 951, 1991.

7. Overmyer RH., 1998.

8. Source: American Heart Association.

## Chapter Two

1. Jeppesen J, et al. Triglyceride concentration and ischemic heart disease: An eight-year follow-up in the Copenhagen Male Study. *Circulation* 97:1029–1036, 1998.

2. Castelli WP, et al. Incidence of coronary heart disease and lipoprotein cholesterol levels. *JAMA* 256: 2835–2838.1986.

3. Stamler J, et. al. Is relationship between serum cholesterol and risk of premature death from coronary heart disease continuous and graded? Findings in 356,222 primary screenees of the Multiple Risk Factor Intervention Trial (MRFIT). *JAMA* 256: 2823–2828, 1986.

4. Rossouw JE, et al. The value of lowering cholesterol after myocardial infarction. *N Engl J Med.* 323: 1112–1119, 1990.

5. Fowkes FGR, et al. Targeting subclinical atherosclerosis. *British Medical Journal* 316: 7147–1764, Jun 13, 1998.

## Chapter Three

1. Second Report of the Expert Panel on Detection, Evaluation, and Treatment of High Blood Cholesterol in Adults (Adult Treatment Panel II). National Cholesterol Education Program Expert Panel. *Circulation* 89: 1329–1445, 1994.

2. Garber AM, et al., Cholesterol screening in asymptomatic adults, revisited. *Ann Int Med.* 124: 518–531, 1996.

3. Scandinavian Simvastatin Survival Study Group. Randomised trial of cholesterol lowering in 4444 patients with coronary heart disease: the Scandinavian Simvastatin Survival Study (4S). *Lancet* 344: 1383–1389, 1994.

4. Sacks FM, et al. The effect of pravastatin on coronary events after myocardial infarction in patients with average cholesterol levels. *N Engl J Med* 335: 1001–1009, 1996.

# Chapter Four

1. Amsterdam EA, et al. Non-pharmacologic therapy for coronary artery atherosclerosis: Results of primary and secondary prevention trials. *Am Heart J* 128: 1344–1352, 1994.

2. Ornish D, et al. Can lifestyle changes reverse coronary heart disease? The Lifestyle Heart Trial. *Lancet* 336: 129–133, 1990; Ornish D, et al. Intensive lifestyle changes for reversal of coronary heart disease. *JAMA* 280: 2001–2007, 1998.

3. Knopp RH, et al. Long-term cholesterol-lowering effects of 4 fat-restricted diets in hypercholesterolemic and combined hyperlipidemic men. The Dietary Alternatives Study. *JAMA* 278 (18): 1509–1515, 1997; Lichtenstein AH, et al. Very low fat diets. *Circulation* 98 (9): 935–939, Sep 1, 1998.

4. Keys A, et al. Serum cholesterol response to changes in the diet, IV: particular saturated fatty acids in the diet. *Metabolism 14:* 776–787, 1965. Hegsted DM, et al. Quantitative effects of dietary fat on serum cholesterol in man. *Am J Clin Nutr.* 17: 281–295, 1965.

5. Temple NJ. Dietary fats and coronary heart disease. *Biomed Pharmacother* 50 (67): 261–268, 1996; Ascherio A, Willett WC. New directions in dietary studies of coronary heart disease. *J Nutr* 125 (3 Suppl): 647S–655S, Mar 1995; Mensink RP, Katan MB. Effect of a diet enriched with monounsaturated or polyunsaturated fatty acids on levels of low-density and high-density lipoprotein in healthy women and men. *N Engl J Med.* 321: 436–441, 1989; Dreon DM, et al. The effects of polyunsaturated fat vs monounsaturated fat on plasma lipoproteins. *JAMA* 263: 2462–2466, 1990; Ginsberg HN, et al. Reduction of plasma cholesterol levels in normal men on an American Heart Association Step I diet or a Step II diet with added monounsaturated fat. *N Engl J Med.* 322: 574–579, 1990.

6. Trichopoulou A, Lagiou P. Worldwide patterns of dietary lipids intake and health implications. *Am J Clin Nutr* 66 (4 Suppl): 961S–964S, Oct 1997.

7. Trichopoulou A, Lagiou P., 1997.

8. Stamler J, Shekelle R. Dietary cholesterol and human coronary heart disease: the epidemiologic evidence. *Arch Pathol Lab Med* 112: 1032–1040, 1988; Shekelle RB, et al. Diet, serum cholesterol, and death from coronary heart disease: the Western Electric study. *N Engl J Med* 304: 65–70, 1981; Kushi LH, et al. Diet and 20-year mortality from coronary heart disease: The Ireland-Boston diet–heart study. *N Engl J Med* 312: 811–818, 1985.

9. Connor WE, et al. N-3 fatty acids from fish oil: effects on plasma lipoproteins and hypertriglyceridemic patients. *Ann N Y Acad Sci* 638: 1634, 1993.

10. Feldman EB, et al. ASCN/AIN Task Force on Trans Fatty Acids of the American Society for Clinical Nutrition and American Institute of Nutrition. Position paper on trans fatty acids. *Am J Clin Nutr* 63: 663–670, 1996; Report of the Expert Panel on Trans Fatty Acids and Coronary Heart Disease. Trans fatty acids and coronary heart disease risk. *Am J Clin Nutr.* 62 (Suppl): 655S–708S, 1995.

11. Butter or margarine? *Harvard Heart Letter* 8: 2, 1–4, Oct 1997.

12. Bell LP, et al. Cholesterol-effects of soluble-fiber cereals as part of a prudent diet for patients with mild to moderate hypercholesterolemia. *Am J Clin Nutr.* 52: 1020–1026, 1990; Whyte JL, et al. Oat bran lowers plasma cholesterol levels in mildly hypercholesterolemic men. *J Am Diet Assoc* 92: 446–449, 1992; Ripsin CM, et al. Oat products and lipid lowering: a meta-analysis. *JAMA* 267: 3317–3325, 1992; Correction in *JAMA* 268: 3074, 1992; Glore SR, et al. Soluble fiber and serum lipids: a literature review. *J Am Diet Assoc* 94: 425–436, 1994.

13. Kritchevsky D. Dietary fibre and cancer. *Eur J Cancer Prev* 6 (5): 435–441, Oct 1997; Liebman, B. Fiber. *Nutrition Action Health Letter* 21: 7, 1–4, Sep. 1994.

14. Rimm EB, et al. Vegetable, fruit, and cereal fiber intake and risk of coronary heart disease among men. *JAMA* 275 (6): 447–451, 1996.

15. Powell KE, et al. Physical activity and the incidence of coronary heart disease. *Annu Rev Public Health* 8: 253–287, 1987; Morris JN, et al. Exercise in leisure time: coronary attack and death rates. *Br Heart J.* 63: 325–334, 1990; Blair SN, et al. Physical fitness and all-cause mortality: a prospective study of healthy men and women. *JAMA* 262: 2395–2401, 1989; Lee IM, Hsieh CC, Paffenbarger RS, Jr. Exercise intensity and longevity in men: the Harvard Alumni Health Study. *JAMA* 273: 1179–1184, 1995.

16. Morris CK, Froelicher VF. Cardiovascular benefits of physical activity. *Herz.*16: 222–236, 1991; Chandrashekhar Y, Anand IS. Exercise as a coronary protective factor. *Am Heart J.* 122: 1723–1739, 1991; Smith SC Jr, et al., and the Secondary Prevention Panel. Preventing heart attack and death in patients with coronary disease. *Circulation* 92: 2–4, 1995.

17. Wenger NK, et al. Cardiac Rehabilitation as Secondary Prevention. Clinical Practice Guideline No. 17. US Department of Health and Human Services, Public Health Service, Agency for Health Care Policy and Research and the National Heart, Lung, and Blood Institute, Rockville, MD, ACHCPR Publication No. 96-0672, October 1995.

18. Blair SN, et al. Physical fitness and all-cause mortality: a prospective study of healthy men and women. *JAMA* 262: 2395–2401, 1989; Lemaitre RN, et al. Leisure-time physical activity and the risk of nonfatal myocardial infarction

in postmenopausal women. *Arch Intern Med.* 155: 2302–2308, 1995.

19. Hagberg JM, et al. Effect of exercise training in 60- to 69-year-old persons with essential hypertension. *Am J Cardiol.* 64: 348–353, 1989; Jennings GL, et al. Exercise, cardiovascular disease and blood pressure. *Clin Exp Hypertens* [A] 11: 1035–1052, 1989; Braith RW, et al. Moderate- and high-intensity exercise lowers blood pressure in normotensive subjects 60 to 79 years of age. *Am J Cardiol* 73: 1124–1128, 1994.

20. Godsland IF, et al. Associations of smoking, alcohol and physical activity with risk factors for coronary heart disease and diabetes in the first follow-up cohort of the Heart Disease and Diabetes Risk Indicators in a Screened Cohort study (HDDRISC-1). *J Intern Med* 244 (1): 33–41, Jul 1998.

21. Ryan C. Hypertension in the elderly patient. *Am Heart J* 122 (4 Pt 2): 1225–1227, Oct 1991.

22. Schuler G, et al. Myocardial perfusion and regression of coronary artery disease in patients on a regimen of intensive physical exercise and low fat diet. *J Am Coll Cardiol.* 19: 34–42, 1992; Schuler G, et al. Regular physical exercise and low-fat diet: effects on progression of coronary artery disease. *Circulation* 86: 1–11, 1992; Haskell WL, et al. Effects of intensive multiple risk factor reduction on coronary atherosclerosis and clinical cardiac events in men and women with coronary artery disease: the Stanford Coronary Risk Intervention Project (SCRIP). *Circulation* 89: 975–990, 1994; Ornish D, et al. Can lifestyle changes reverse coronary heart disease? The Lifestyle Heart Trial. *Lancet* 336: 129–133, 1990.

23. Dishman RK. Compliance/adherence in health related exercise. *Health Psychol* 1: 237–267, 1982.

24. Hills AP, Byrne NM. Exercise prescription for weight management. *Proc Nutr Soc* 57 (1): 93–103, Feb 1998; Pinto BM, Szymanski L. Exercise in weight management. *Med Health R I* 80 (11):361–363, Nov 1997.

25. Stunkard AJ. Current views on obesity. *Am J Med.* 100: 230–236, 1996.

26. Blair SN. Evidence for success of exercise in weight loss and control. *Ann Intern Med.* 119: 702–706, 1993; Grilo CM. Physical activity and obesity. *Biomed Pharmacother.* 48: 127–136, 1994.

27. Blackburn G. Effect of degree of weight loss on health benefits. *Obes Res* 3 (suppl 2): 211s–216s, 1995; Goldstein DJ. Beneficial health effects of modest weight loss. *Int J Obes Relat Metab Disord* 16: 397–415, 1992.

28. *Harvard Heart Letter* 8: 6, 1–4, Feb 1998.

29. Klatsky AL, et al. Alcohol and mortality. *Ann Intern Med.* 117: 646–654, 1992. Steinberg D, et al. Alcohol and atherosclerosis. *Ann Intern Med.* 114: 967–976, 1991.

30. Thun MJ, et al. Alcohol consumption and mortality among middle-aged and elderly U.S. adults. *N Engl J Med* 337(24): 1705–1714, 1997.

31. Beer aids the heart, too. *Australian Nursing Journal* 5: 6, 15, Dec 1997–Jan 1998.

32. Kawachi K, et al. Does coffee drinking increase the risk of coronary heart disease? Results from a meta-analysis. *Br Heart J* 72: 269–275, 1994.

33. Willett WC, et al. Coffee consumption and coronary heart disease in women. A ten-year follow-up. *JAMA* 275 (6): 458–462, 1996; Schwarz B, et al. Coffee, tea and lifestyle. *Prev Med* 23: 377–384, 1994.

34. Dhond M, Amserdam EA. Secondary prevention therapy in patients with coronary artery disease. *Formulary* 33: 120–136, 1998.

35. Dhond M, Amserdam EA., 1998.

36. Scandinavian Simvastatin Survival Study Group., 1994.

37. Sacks FM, et al., 1996.

38. Hoogerbrugge N, et al. Estrogen replacement decreases the level of antibodies against oxidized low-density lipo-protein in postmenopausal women with coronary heart disease. *Metabolism* 47 (6): 675–680, Jun 1998.

39. Wren BG. Megatrials of hormonal replacement therapy. *Drugs Aging* 12 (5): 343–348, May 1998.

40. Barrett-Connor E, Grady D. Hormone replacement therapy, heart disease, and other considerations. *Annu Rev Public Health* 19: 55–72, 1998.

41. Dhond M, Amserdam EA., 1998.

## Chapter Five

1. Covington R, ed. Handbook of nonprescription drugs. American Pharmaceutical Association, 373–374, 1996.

2. Conner PI, et al. Fifteen-year mortality in Coronary Drug Project patients: long-term benefit with niacin. *J Am Coll Cardiol* 8: 1245–1255, 1986.

3. Ginsberg HN, Goldberg IJ. Harrison's PIM CD-ROM. Endocrinology and Metabolism, 341; Disorders of Lipo-protein Metabolism—Diagnosis. Part Thirteen, 1998.

4. McKenney JM, et al. A comparison of the efficacy and toxic effects of sustained- vs. immediate-release niacin in

hypercholesterolemic patients. *JAMA* 271: 672–677, 1994; Christensen AN, et al. Nicotinic acid treatment of hypercholesterolemia. *JAMA* 177: 546–550, 1961; Knopp RH, et al. Contrasting effects of unmodified and time-release forms of niacin on lipoproteinis in hyperlipidemia subjects: clues to mechanism of action of niacin. *Metabolism* 34: 642–650, 1985; Superko HR, Krauss RM. Differential effects of nicotinic acid in subjects with different LDL subclass patterns. *Atherosclerosis* 95: 69–76, 1992.

5. Covington R, ed., 1996.

6. Head, KA. Inositol hexaniacinate: A safer alternative to niacin. *Alt Med Rev* 1: 176–184, 1996.

7. Wyandt CM, Williamson JS. Vitamins: What the pharmacist should know. *Drug Topics*: 74–83, Jul 21, 1997.

8. Jungnickel PW, et al. Effect of two aspirin pretreatment regimens on niacin-induced cutaneous reactions. *J Gen Intern Med* 12: 591–596. October 1997.

9. McKenney JM, et al., 1994.

10. Ginsberg HN, Goldberg IJ., 1998.

11. Clementz GI, Holmes AW. Nicotinic acid-induced fulminant hepatic failure. *J Clin Gastroenterol.* 9: 582–584, 1987.

12. Rader JI, et al. Hepatic toxicity of unmodified and time-release preparations of niacin. *Am J Med.* 92: 77–81, 1992.

13. Knopp RH, et al. Contrasting effects of unmodified and time-release forms of niacin on lipoproteinis in hyperlipidemia subjects: clues to mechanism of action of niacin. *Metabolism* 34: 642–650, 1985; Superko HR, Krauss RM. Differential effects of nicotinic acid in subjects with different LDL subclass patterns. *Atherosclerosis* 95: 69–76, 1992.

14. McKenney JM, et al., 1994.

15. Ginsberg HN, Goldberg IJ., 1998.


# Chapter Six

1. Elnima EL, et al. The antimicrobial activity of garlic and onion extracts. *Pharmazie* 38: 747–748, 1983.

2. Silagy CA, et al. A meta-analysis of the effect of garlic on blood pressure. *J Hypertens* 12(4): 463–468, 1994.

3. Kamanna VS, et al. Effect of garlic (*Allium sativum* Linn.) on serum lipoproteins and lipoprotein cholesterol levels in Albino rats rendered hypercholesteremic by feeding cholesterol. *Lipids* 17: 438, 1982; Lau B, et al. *Allium sativum* (garlic) and cancer prevention. *Nutr Res* 10: 937–948, 1990.

4. Bordia A, et al. Effect of essential oil of onion and garlic on experimental atherosclerosis in rabbits. *Atherosclerosis* 26: 379–386, 1977; Efendi JL, et al. The effect of the aged garlic extract, "Kyolic," on the development of experimental atherosclerosis. *Atherosclerosis* 132(1): 37–42, 1997; Heinle H, et al. Effects of dietary garlic supplementation in a rat model of atherosclerosis. *Arzneim-Forsch/Drug Res* 44: 614–617, 1994; Jain RC, et al. Effect of garlic oil in experimental cholesterol atherosclerosis. *Atherosclerosis* 29: 125–129, 1978; Schulz V, et al. Rational phytotherapy. New York: Springer-Verlag, pp. 112–113, 115, 121, 1998.

5. Mader FH, Treatment of hyperlipidaemia with garlic-powder tablets. Evidence from the German Association of General Practitioners' multicentric placebo-controlled double-blind study. *Arzneimittelforschung* 40(10): 1111–1116, 1990.

6. Adesh K, et al. Can Garlic reduce levels of serum lipids? A controlled clinical study. *Am J Med* 94: 632–635, 1993.

7. Silagy CA, et al. A meta-analysis of the effect of garlic on blood pressure. *J Hypertens* 12(4): 463–468, 1994.

8. Neil HA, et al. Garlic powder in the treatment of moderate hyperlipidaemia: A controlled trial and meta-analysis. *J R Coll Physicians Lond* 30(4): 329–334, 1996.

9. Steiner M, et al. A double-blind crossover study in moderately hypercholesterolemic men that compared the effect of aged garlic extract and placebo administration on blood lipids. *Am J Clin Nutr* 64(6): 866–870, 1996.

10. Berthold HK, et al. Effect of a garlic oil preparation on serum lipoproteins and cholesterol metabolism. A Randomized Controlled Trial *JAMA* 279: 1900–1902, 1998; Santos O S De A, et al. Effects of garlic powder and garlic oil preparations on blood lipids, blood pressure and well-being. *Br J of Clin Res* 6: 91–100, 1995.

11. Breithaupt-Grogler K, et al. Protective effect of chronic garlic intake on the elastic properties of the aorta in the elderly. *Circulation* 96(7): 2749–2655, 1997.

12. Bordia A, Knoblauch und koronare Herzkrankheit: Wirkungen einer dreijahrigen Behandlung mit Knoblauchextrakt auf die Reinfarkt-und Mortalitatsrate. *Dtsch Apoth Ztg* 129 (Suppl 15): 16–17, 1989; Reported in the European Scientific Cooperative on Phytotherapy Monographs Fascicule 3, *Allii sativi* bulbus (Garlic) p4, ESCOP, Exeter, UK, 1997.

13. Popov I, et al. Antioxidant effects of aqueous garlic extract, 1st communication: direct detection using photochemo-luminescence. *Arzneimittelforschung Drug*

*Res* 44(1): 602–604, 1994; Prasad K, et al. Antioxidant activity of allicin, an active principle in garlic. *Mol Cell Biochem* 148(2): 183–189, 1995; Torok B, et al. Effectiveness of garlic on radical activity in radical generating systems. *Arzneimittelforschung Drug Res* 44(1): 608–611, 1994.

14. Breithaupt-Grogler K, et al., 1997.

15. Gebhardt R, Multiple inhibitory effects of garlic extracts on cholesterol biosynthesis in hepatocytes. *Lipids* 28(6): 613–619, 1993; Gebhardt R, et al. Inhibition of cholesterol biosynthesis by allicin and ajoene in rat hepatocytes and HepG2 cells. *Biochem Biophys Acta* 1213: 57–62, 1994; Gebhardt R, et al. Differential inhibitory effects of garlic-derived organosulfur compounds on cholesterol biosynthesis in primary rat hepatocyte cultures. *Lipids* 31(12): 1269–1276, 1996; Quereshi AA, et al. Inhibition of cholesterol and fatty acid biosynthesis in liver enzymes and chicken hepatocytes by polar fractions of garlic. *Lipids* 18: 343–348, 1983.

16. Lawson LD, et al. Identification and HPLC quantitation(sic) of the sulfides and dialk(en)yl thiosulfinates in commercial garlic products. *Planta Med* 57: 363–370, 1991.

17. Sumiyoshi H, et al. Chronic toxicity test of garlic extracts in rats. *J Toxicol Sci* 9: 61–75, 1984.

18. Abraham SK, et al. Genotoxicity of garlic, turmeric, and asafoetida in mice. *Mutat Res* 136: 85–88, 1984; Yoshida S, et al. Mutagenicity and cytotoxicity tests of garlic. *J Toxicol Sci* 9: 77–86, 1984.

19. Schulz V, et al. Rational phytotherapy. New York: Springer-Verlag, pp. 112–113, 115, 121, 1998.

20. Schulz V, et al., 1998.

## Chapter Seven

1. Anderson JW, Johnstone BM, Cook-Newell ME. Meta-analysis of the effects of soy protein intake on serum lipids. *N Engl J Med* 333: 276–282, 1995.

   Cline JM, et al. Phytochemicals for the prevention of breast and endometrial cancer. *Cancer Treat Res.* 94: 107–134, 1998.

2. Messina MJ, et al. Soy intake and cancer risk: a review of the in vitro and in vivo data. *Nutr Cancer* 21(2): 113–131, 1994.

3. Miettinen TA, et al. Reduction of serum cholesterol with sitostanol-ester margarine in a mildly hypercholesterolemic population. *N Engl J Med* 16, 333 (20): 1308–1312, Nov 1995.

4. Heber, D. et al. Cholesterol lowering effects of a proprietary Chinese red yeast rice dietary supplement. *FASEB Journal* 12(4): A206, 1998.

5. Chang M. Cholestin: Healthcare professional product guide. Pharmanex: Simi Valley, CA, 1–6, 1998.

6. Parker RA, et al. Tocotrienols regulate cholesterol production in mammalian cells by post-transcriptional suppression of 3-hydroxy-3-methylglutaryl-coenzyme A reductase. *J Biol Chem* 25, 268 (15): 11230–11238, May 1993; Pearce BC, et al. Hypocholesterolemic activity of synthetic and natural tocotrienols. *J Med Chem* 2, 35 (20): 3595–3606, Oct 1992.

7. Qureshi AA, et al. Novel tocotrienols of rice bran modulate cardiovascular disease risk parameters of hypercholesterolemic humans. *J Nutrit Biochem* 8: 290–298, 1997.

8. Tomeo AC, et al. Antioxidant effects of tocotrienols in patients with hyperlipidemia and carotid stenosis. *Lipids* 30 (12): 1179–1183, Dec 1995.

9. Kromhout D, et al. Alcohol, fish, fibre and antioxidant vitamins intake do not explain population differences in coronary heart disease mortality. *Int J Epidemiol* 25: 753–759, 1996; Dyerberg, J. n- 3 Fatty Acids and coronary artery disease. potentials and problems. *Omega-3, Lipoproteins and Atherosclerosis* 27: 251–258, 1996.

10. Harris WS. n-3 Fatty acids and serum lipoproteins: human studies. *Am J Clin Nutr* 65 (suppl): 1645S–1654S, 1997.

11. Dyerberg J. n- 3 Fatty Acids and coronary artery disease. potentials and problems. *Omega-3, Lipoproteins and Atherosclerosis* 27: 251–258, 1996.

12. Prichard BN, et al. Fish oils and cardiovascular disease. *BMJ* 310: 819–820, 1995. Stone NJ. From the Nutrition Committee of the American Heart Association. Fish consumption, fish oil, lipids, and coronary heart disease. *Am J Clin Nutr* 65: 1083–1086, 1997.

13. Pietinen P, et al. Intake of fatty acids and risk of coronary heart disease in a cohort of Finnish men: the alpha-tocopherol, beta-carotene cancer prevention study. *Am J Epidemiol* 145 (10): 876–887, 1997.

14. Harris WS. Dietary fish oil and blood lipids. *Curr Opin Lipidol* 7: 3–7, 1996.

15. Harris WS., 1997.

16. Laurora G, et al. Delayed arteriosclerosis progression in high risk subjects treated with mesoglycan. Evaluation of intima-media thickness. *J Cardiovasc Surg* (Torino) 34 (4): 313–318, 1993; Tanganelli P, et al. Updating on in-vivo and in-vitro effects of heparin and other glycosaminoglycans (mesoglycan) on arterial endothelium: a morphometrical study. *Int J Tissue React* 14 (3): 149–153, 1992.

17. Gaddi A, et al. Controlled evaluation of pantethine, a natural hypolipidemic compound, in patients with different forms of hyperlipoproteinemia. *Atherosclerosis* 50 (1): 73–83, 1984; Rubba R, Postiglione A, DeSimone B, et al. Comparative evaluation of the lipid-lowering effects of fenofibrate and pantethine in type II hyperlipoproteinemia. *Curr Ther Res Clin Exp* 38: 719–727, 1985; Angelico M et al. Improvement in serum lipid profile in hyper-lipoproteinaemic patients after treatment with pantethine: a crossover, double-blind trial versus placebo. *Curr Ther Res* 33:1091, 1983.

18. Agarwal RC, et al. Clinical trial of gugulipid a new hyperlipidemic agent of plant origin in primary hyperlipidemia. *Indian J Med Res* 84, 626–634, 1986; Nityanand, S, et al. Clinical trials with gugulipid. A new hypolipidaemic agent. *J Assoc Physicians India* 37 (5): 323–328, 1989.

19. Mertz W. Chromium in human nutrition: a review. *J Nutr* 123 (4): 626–633, April 1993.

20. Davini P, et al. Controlled study on L-carnitine therapeutic efficacy in post-infarction. *Drugs Exp Clin Res* 18 (8): 355–365, 1992.

21. Bell L, et al. Cholesterol-lowering effects of calcium carbonate in patients with mild to moderate hypercholesterolemia. *Arch Intern Med* 152: 2441–2444, 1992.

22. Oosthuizen W, et al. Lecithin has no effect on serum lipoprotein, plasma fibrinogen and macro molecular protein complex levels in hyperlipidaemic men in a double-blind controlled study. *Eur J Clin Nutr* 52 (6): 419–424, Jun 1998.

## Chapter Eight

1. Covington R, ed. Handbook of nonprescription drugs. American Pharmaceutical Association: 369–370, 1996.

2. Stephens NG, et al. Randomised controlled trial of vitamin E in patients with coronary disease: Cambridge Heart Antioxidant Study (CHAOS). *Lancet* 347: 781–786, 1996.

3. Rimm EB, et al. Vitamin E consumption and the risk of coronary heart disease in men. *N Engl J Med* 328 (20): 1450–1456, 1993.

4. Manson JE, et al. A prospective study of antioxidant vitamins and incidence of coronary heart disease in women. Abstract. *J Am Coll Nutr* 11 (5): 609, 1992; Stampfer M, et al. Vitamin E consumption and the risk of coronary heart disease in women. *N Engl J Med* 328: 1444–1449, 1993.

5. Losonczy KG, et al. Vitamin E and vitamin C supplement use and risk of all-cause and coronary heart disease mortality in older persons: the Established Populations for Epidemiologic Studies of the Elderly. *Am J Clin Nutr* 64: 190–196, 1996.

6. Gey KF. Vitamins E plus C and interacting conutrients required for optimal health. A critical and constructive review of epidemiology and supplementation data regarding cardiovascular disease and cancer. *Biofactors* 7 (1–2): 113–174, 1998.

7. Rapola JM, et al. Randomised trial of a-tocopherol and b-carotene supplements on incidence of major coronary events in men with previous myocardial infarction. *Lancet* 349: 1715–1720, 1997; Rapola JM, et al. Effect of vitamin E and beta-carotene on the incidence of angina pectoris. *JAMA* 275: 693–698, 1996; Albanes D, et al. Effects of alpha-tocopherol and beta-carotene supplements on cancer incidence in the Alpha-Tocopherol Beta-Carotene Cancer Prevention Study. *Am J Clin Nutr* 62 (suppl): 1427S–1430S, 1995.

8. Jialal I, Fuller CJ. Effect of vitamin E, vitamin C and beta-carotene on LDL oxidation and atherosclerosis. *Can J Cardiol* 1 (Suppl G): 97G–103G, 1995; Goshman L. Vitamin E and coronary artery disease. Center for Drug Policy and Clinical Economics, Univ. of Wisconsin Hospital and Clinics, May 1996; Stephens NG, et al. Randomised controlled trial of vitamin E in patients with coronary disease: Cambridge Heart Antioxidant Study (CHAOS). *Lancet* 347: 781–786, 1996.

9. Morel DW, De la Llera-Moya M, Friday KE. Treatment of cholesterol-fed rabbits with dietary vitamins E and C inhibits lipoprotein oxidation but not development of atherosclerosis. *J Nutr* 124: 2123–2130, 1994.

10. Calzada C, et al. The influence of antioxidant nutrients on platelet function in healthy volunteers. *Atherosclerosis* 128 (1) : 97–105, 1997.

11. Rimm EB, Stampfer MJ. The role of antioxidants in preventive cardiology. *Curr Opin Cardiol* 12 (2): 188–194, March 1997.

12. Longo D. Part five—Nutrition. Harrison's Principles of Internal Medicine 14/e. CD-ROM. New York: McGraw-Hill, 1998.

13. Kiyose C, et al. Biodiscrimination of alpha-tocopherol stereoisomers in humans after oral administration. *Am J Clin Nutr* 65(3): 785–789, 1997.

14. Burton GW, et al. Human plasma and tissue alpha-tocopherol concentrations in response to supplementation with deuterated natural and synthetic vitamin E. *Am J Clin Nutr* 67(4): 669–684, 1998.

15. Christen S, et al. Gamma-tocopherol traps mutagenic electrophiles such as NOX and complements alpha-tocopherol: physiological implications, *Proc Natl Acad Sci USA* 94: 3217–3222, 1997.

16. Longo D, 1998.

17. Covington R, ed., 1996.

18. Albanes D, et al. Effects of alpha-tocopherol and beta-carotene supplements on cancer incidence in the Alpha-Tocopherol Beta-Carotene Cancer Prevention Study. *Am J Clin Nutr* 62 (suppl): 1427S–1430S, 1995.

19. Steiner M, et al. Vitamin E plus aspirin compared with aspirin alone in patients with transient ischemic attacks. *Am J Clin Nutr* 62 (suppl): 1381S–1384S, 1995.

20. Covington R, ed., 370–372, 1996.

21. Ness AR. Vitamin C and cardiovascular disease. *Nutrition Report* 15 (3), May/Jun 1997; Simon JA. Vitamin C and cardiovascular disease: a review. *J Am Coll Nutr* 11 (2): 107–125, 1992; Trout DL. Vitamin C and cardiovascular risk factors. *Am J Clin Nutr* 53: 322S–325S, 1991.

22. Losonczy KG, et al. Vitamin E and vitamin C supplement use and risk of all-cause and coronary heart disease mortality in older persons: the Established Populations for Epidemiologic Studies of the Elderly. *Am J Clin Nutr* 64: 190–196, 1996.

23. Gey KF. Vitamins E plus C and interacting co-nutrients required for optimal health. A critical and constructive review of epidemiology and supplementation data regarding cardiovascular disease and cancer. *Biofactors* 7 (1–2): 113–174, 1998.

24. Covington R, ed., 1996.

25. Levine M, et al., *Proceedings of the National Academy of Sciences* 93 (8): 3704–3709, April 16, 1996.

26. Covington R, ed., 1996.

27. Gerster H. No contribution of ascorbic acid to renal calcium oxalate stones. *Ann Nutr Metab* 41(5): 269–282, 1997.

28. Kohlmeier L, Hastings SB. Epidemiologic evidence of a role of carotenoids in cardiovascular disease prevention. *Am J Clin Nutr* 62 (suppl): 1370S–1376S, 1995. Reunanen A, et al. Antioxidant vitamin intake and coronary mortality in an longitudinal population study. *Am J Epidemiol* 139: 1180–1189, 1994.

29. Albanes D, et al. Alpha-tocopherol, Beta-carotene Cancer Prevention Study Group. The effect of vitamin E and beta-carotene on the incidence of lung cancer and other cancers in male smokers. *N Engl J Med* 330: 1029–1035, 1994.

30. Rapola JM, et al. Randomised trial of a-tocopherol and b-carotene supplements on incidence of major coronary events in men with previous myocardial infarction. *Lancet* 349: 1715–1720, 1997.

31. Rapola JM, et al. Effect of vitamin E and beta carotene on the incidence of angina pectoris. *JAMA* 275 (9): 693–698, 1996.

32. White WS, et al. Pharmacokinetics of beta-carotene and canthaxanthin after individual and combined doses by human subjects. *J Am Coll Nutr* 13: 665–671, 1994.

33. Longo D, 1998; Heywood R, et al., The toxicity of beta-carotene. *Toxicology* 36, 91–100, 1985.

## Chapter Nine

1. Graham IM, et al. Plasma homocysteine as a risk factor for vascular disease. The European Concerted Action Project. *JAMA* 277: 1775–1781, 1997.

2. Aronow WS, Ahn C. Association between plasma homocysteine and coronary artery disease in older persons. *Am J Cardiol* 80 (9):1216–1218, Nov 1, 1997; Graham IM, et al. Plasma homocysteine as a risk factor for vascular disease.

The European Concerted Action Project. *JAMA* 277: 1775–1781, 1997.

3. Nygard O, et al. Plasma homocysteine levels and mortality in patients with coronary artery disease. *N Engl J Med.* 337 (4): 230–236, Jul 24, 1997.

4. Folsom AR, et al. Prospective study of coronary heart disease incidence in relation to fasting total homocysteine, related genetic polymorphisms, and B vitamins: the Atherosclerosis Risk in Communities (ARIC) study. *Circulation* 98 (3): 204–210, Jul 21, 1998.

## Chapter Ten

1. Moghadasian MH, et al. Homocysteine and coronary artery disease. *Arch Intern Med* 157: 2299–2308, 1997.

2. Ubbink JB, et al. Hyperhomocysteinemia and the response to vitamin supplementation. *Clin Investig* 71 (12): 993–998, Dec 1993.

3. Rimm EB, et al. Folate and vitamin $B_6$ from diet and supplements in relation to risk of coronary heart disease among women. *JAMA* 279 (5): 359–364, 1998.

4. Rimm EB, et al., 1998.

5. Covington R, ed. Handbook of nonprescription drugs. American Pharmaceutical Association: 372–373, 1996.

6. Covington R, ed., 1996.

7. Rimm EB, et al., 1998.

8. Ballal RS, et al. Homocysteine: update on a new risk factor. *Cleve Clin J Med* 64: 543–549, 1997.

9. Fallest-Strobl PC, et al. Homocysteine: a new risk factor for atherosclerosis. *Am Fam Physician* 56: 1607–1612, 1997.

10. Ballal RS, et al., 1997.

11. Covington R, ed., 1996.

12. Campbell NR. How safe are folic acid supplements? *Arch Intern Med* 156: 1638–1644, 1996.

13. Covington R, ed., 1996.

14. Covington R, ed., p 375, 1996.

15. Saltzman JR, et al. Effect of hypochlorhydria due to omeprazole treatment or atrophic gastritis on protein-bound $B_{12}$ absorption. *J Am Coll Nutr* 13 (6): 584–591, 1994; Van Goor, et al. Review. Cobalamin deficiency and mental impairment in elderly people. *Age Ageing*, 24: 536–542, 1995.

## Chapter Twelve

1. Joint National Committee on Prevention, Detection, Evaluation, and Treatment of High Blood Pressure. The sixth report of the Joint National Committee on Prevention, Detection, Evaluation, and Treatment of High Blood Pressure (JNC VI). *Arch Intern Med* 157: 2413–2446, 1997.

2. Nurminen ML, et al. Dietary factors in the pathogenesis and treatment of hypertension. *Ann Med* 30 (2): 143–150, Apr 1998.

3. Joint National Committee on Prevention, Detection, Evaluation, and Treatment of High Blood Pressure, 1997.

4. Appel LJ, et al. A clinical trial of the effects of dietary patterns on blood pressure. *N Engl J Med.* 336: 1117–1124, 1997.

5. Joint National Committee on Prevention, Detection, Evaluation, and Treatment of High Blood Pressure, 1997.

6. Joint National Committee on Prevention, Detection, Evaluation, and Treatment of High Blood Pressure., 1997.

7. Joint National Committee on Prevention, Detection, Evaluation, and Treatment of High Blood Pressure. The sixth report of the Joint National Committee on Prevention, Detection, Evaluation, and Treatment of High Blood Pressure (JNC VI). *Arch Intern Med* 153: 154–183, 1993.

8. Joint National Committee on Prevention, Detection, Evaluation, and Treatment of High Blood Pressure., 1997.

9. Hixson KA, et al. The relation between religiosity, selected health behaviors, and blood pressure among adult females. *Prev Med* 27 (4): 545–552, Jul 1998.

10. Hansson L, et al. The Captoril Prevention Project (CAPPP) in hypertension-baseline data and current status. *Blood Pressure* 6: 365–367, 1997.

## Chapter Thirteen

1. Nurminen ML, et al. Dietary factors in the pathogenesis and treatment of hypertension. *Ann Med* 30 (2): 143–150, Apr 1998.

2. Joint National Committee on Prevention, Detection, Evaluation, and Treatment of High Blood Pressure, 1997.

3. Whelton PK, et al. Effects of oral potassium on blood pressure. Meta-analysis of randomized controlled clinical trials. *JAMA* 277(20): 1624–1632, 1997.

4. Altura BM, et al. Magnesium, hypertensive vascular diseases, atherogenesis, subcellular compartmentation of $Ca^{2+}$ and $Mg^{2+}$ and vascular contractility. *Miner Electrolyte Metab* 19 (4–5): 323–336, 1993.

5. Kawano Y, et al. Effects of magnesium supplementation in hypertensive patients: assessment by office, home, and ambulatory blood pressures. *Hypertension* 32 (2): 260–265, Aug 1998; Yamamoto ME, et al. Lack of blood pressure effect with calcium and magnesium supplementation in adults with high-normal blood pressure. Results from Phase I of the Trials of Hypertension Prevention (TOHP). Trials of Hypertension Prevention (TOHP) Collaborative Research Group. *Ann Epidemiol* 5 (2): 96–107, Mar 1995; Mizushima S, Dietary magnesium intake and blood pressure: a qualitative overview of the observational studies. *J Hum Hypertens* 12 (7): 447–453, Jul 1998.

6. Hatton DC, McCarron DA. Dietary calcium and blood pressure in experimental models of hypertension: a review. *Hypertension* 23 (4): 513–530, Apr 1994.

7. Bucher HC, et al. Effects of dietary calcium supplementation on blood pressure. A meta-analysis of randomized controlled trials. *JAMA* 275 (13): 1016–1022, 1996.

8. Weber C, et al. Effect of dietary coenzyme $Q_{10}$ as an antioxidant in human plasma. *Mol Aspects Med* 15 (Suppl.): S97–S102, 1994.

9. Alleva T, et al. The roles of coenzyme $Q_{10}$ and vitamin E on the peroxidation of human low density lipoprotein subfractions. *Proc Natl Acad Sci USA* 92: 9388–9891, 1995.

10. Digiesi V, et al. Effect of coenzyme $Q_{10}$ on essential arterial hypertension. *Curr Ther Res* 47: 841–]845, 1990.

11. Digiesi V, et al. Coenzyme $Q_{10}$ in essential hypertension. *Mol Aspects Med* 15 (Suppl): S257–S263, 1994.

12. Langsjoen PH, et al. Treatment of essential hypertension with coenzyme $Q_{10}$. *Mol Aspects Med* 15 (Suppl.): S265–S272, 1994.

13. Weiss M. Bioavailability of four oral coenzyme $Q_{10}$ formulations in healthy volunteers. *Mol Aspects Med* 15 (Suppl.): S273–S280, 1994.

14. Bargossi AM, et al. Exogenous $CoQ_{10}$ supplementation prevents plasma ubiquinone reduction induced by HMG-CoA reductase inhibitors. *Mol Aspects Med* 15 (Suppl.): S187–S193, 1994.

15. Silagy CA, et al. A meta-analysis of the effect of garlic on blood pressure. *J Hypertens* 12(4): 463–468, 1994.

16. Auer W, et al. Hypertension and hyperlipidemia: garlic helps in mild cases. *Br J Clin Pract Symp* Suppl 69: 3–6, 1990.

17. Santos O S De A, et al. Effects of garlic powder and garlic oil preparations on blood lipids, blood pressure and well-being. *Br J of Clin Res* 6: 91–100, 1995.

18. Appel LJ, et al. Does supplementation of diet with 'fish oil' reduce blood pressure? A meta-analysis of controlled clinical trials. *Arch Intern Med* 153 (12): 1429–1438, 1993.

19. Berry EM, Hirsch. Does dietary linolenic acid influence blood pressure? *Am J Clin Nutr.* 44 (3): 336–340, Sep 1986.

20. Douhan A, et al. Significance of magnesium in congestive heart failure. *Am Heart J* 132: 664–671, 1996.

21. Forster A, et al. Crataegus be massig reduzierter links-ventrikularer Auswurffraktion. Ergospirometrische Verlaufsuntersuchung bei 72 Patienten in doppelblindem Vergleich mit Plazebo. *Munch Med Wochenschr* 136 (Suppl 1): 21–26, 1994. In Shulz V, 97, 1998.

22. Fischer K, et al. Crataegus-Extrakt vs. Methydigoxin. Einfluss auf Rehologie und Mikrozirkulation bei 12 gesunden Probanden. *Munch Med Wochenschr* 136 (Suppl 1): 35–38, 1994. In Shulz V, 90, 1998; Tauchert M,

et al. *Crataegi folium* cum Flore bei Herzinsuffizienz, 1995. In Loew D, Tietbrock N, eds. Phytopharmaka in Forschung und klinischer Anwendung. Darmstadt: Steinkopff Verlag: 137–144. In Shulz V, 95–97, 1998.

23. Schulz V, et al., 1998.

# Index

## A

Ace inhibitors, hypertension, 129–130
Acerola fruit, benefits, 95–96
African Americans
  CAD risk, 11
  heart attack mortality, 7
  hypertension risks, 117
Age, CAD risk, 10
AHA, see American Heart Association
Alcohol
  –beta-carotene, contraindications, 100
  limiting, 47–48
  moderation, definition, 48
Allicin, 67
Alpha-blockers, hypertension, 130–131
Alpha-tocopherol, see Vitamin E
Alzheimer's disease, misdiagnosis, 9
American Heart Association
  dietary recommendations
    fats, 28, 30–31

    fiber, 33–35
    Step I and II diets, 27–29
Angina
  description, 5–6
  hawthorn benefits, 142, 153
  silent, 2
  smokers, beta-carotene risks, 99
  symptoms, 2
  treatments, 6
Angiotensin II receptor blockers, hypertension, 130
Antabuse, see Disulfiram
Antibiotics, garlic as, 67
Anticoagulants
  garlic as, 73
  –garlic, interaction, 73
  –ginkgo, interaction, 73
  –vitamin E, interaction, 93
Anticonvulsants–folic acid interactions, 112
Antioxidants, see also Free radicals
  description, 87
  $CoQ_{10}$ as, 101, 138

Antioxidants (*continued*)
  garlic as, 70, 101
  heart disease and, overview, 149–150
  lipoic acid, 101
  PCOs as, 101
  resveratrol as, 101
  selenium as, 101
  soy as, 101
  tocotrienols as, 79
  turmeric as, 101
Anti-viral, garlic as, 67
Arrhythmia, cause, 2
Ascorbic acid, *see* Vitamin C
Aspirin, for flushing reaction, 61
Asthma, beta-blockers, contraindications, 130
Atherosclerosis
  acceleration, 3
  description, 2
  development, 3
  effects, 2–3
  etymology, 2
  hypertension association, 118–119
  oxidation and, 4–5
  stroke association, 8
Atorvastatin, 49
Atromid-D, 51

**B**
Bacterial infections, 3–4
Baycol, 49
Beans
  fat content, 41
  serving recommendations, 35

Beta-blockers, 130
Beta-carotene
  CAD, 98–100
  description, 97
  dosage, 100
  food sources, 98–99, 100
  as marker, 99–100
  overview, 150
  safety, 100
Bezafibrate, 51
Bilberry, cholesterol-lowering activities, 85
Bile acids, production, 15
Bile acid sequestrants, 51–52
Blood
  clots, *see* Thrombi
  pooling, 8
  pressure, *see also* Hypertension
    classification, 121–122
    diastolic, 116, 122–123
    optimal, 122
    salt sensitivity, 126
    systolic, 116, 122–123
    variation, 116
BMI, *see* Body mass index
Body mass index
  calculating, 46
  description, 45
  hypertension association, 124–125
Breads
  lowfat, 41
  serving recommendations, 35
Breast cancer
  alcohol association, 48
  ERT risks, 53

# C

CAD, *see* Coronary artery
   disease
Caffeine, *see* Coffee
Calcium
   blood pressure–lowering
      effects, 136
   channel-blockers, *see*
      Calcium antagonists
   cholesterol-lowering activity,
      84
   daily value, 137
   in dairy products, 37
   food sources, 137
Calcium antagonists,
   hypertension, 131
Calories, fat, 39
Cancer, *see also specific types*
   prevention
      flax oil, 82
      monounsaturated fats,
         31–32
      red yeast rice, risks, 78
      risks, soy benefits, 76
Canola oil, benefits, 32
Cardiovascular system,
   description, 1
CARE, *see* Cholesterol and
   Recurrent Events Trial
Central nervous system
   degeneration, 88
Cerebrovascular disease,
   description, 2–3
Cerivastatin, 49
CHAOS study, description,
   88–89
CHF, *see* Congestive heart
   failure

Childhood, atherosclerosis in, 3
*Chlamydia,* 3–4
Cholesterol, *see also*
      Dyslipidemias;
      Hypercholesterolemia;
      *specific types*
   benefits, 15
   description, 16
   consuming, 16
   endothelium injury, 4
   home test, 21
   managing high cholesterol,
      *see* Hypercholesterolemia
   plaque build-up by, 15
   types, 16
Cholesterol and Recurrent
   Events Trial, 50–51
Cholestyramine, 51
Chromium, cholesterol-
   lowering activity, 83–84
Cigarette smoking, *see*
   Smoking
Clinical intervention trial,
   description, 58–59
Clofibrate, 51
Coenzyme Q₁₀
   blood pressure–lowering
      activity, 137–138, 152
   CAD, 137–138
   CHF, 137–139
   description, 137–138
   dosage, 139–140
   overview, 152
   safety, 140
   sources, 138
   studies, 138–139
Coffee, 48, 127
Colestid, 51

Colestipol, 51
Collagen formation, 88
Colorectal cancer, 51
Congestive heart failure
  description, 7
  CoQ$_{10}$, 137, 139
  heart attack association, 7–8
  mild, hawthorn benefits,
    142, 153
Coronary artery disease, *see
    also related ailments*
  cause, 3–4
  description, 1–2
  conventional therapies
    angioplasty, 53
    bypass surgery, 53
    diet
      fats, 27–33
      fiber, 33–34
      Food Guide Pyramid,
        35–37
    exercise, 39–43
    weight control, 43–44
  first sign, v
  incidence, vii
  LDL cholesterol association,
    18
  mortality ranking, v
  natural therapies
    beta-carotene, 98–100,
      150
    CoQ$_{10}$, 137–138
    EFAs, 81
    folic acid, 112–113
      studies, 105–109
      therapy, 109–112
    garlic, 66–73
    vitamin B$_6$, 105–109

  vitamin B$_{12}$, 105–109,
    113–114
  vitamin C, 93, 149–150
  vitamin E, 89–92, 149–150
  preventing, overview, 146
  risk factors
    aging, 10
    alcohol, excessive, 48
    cholesterol levels, 11,
      17–18
    coffee, excessive, 48
    diabetes, 12
    gender, 11
    heredity, 11
    homocysteine, 103–105
    hypertension, 11–12
    list, 9–10
    NCEP, 23
    obesity, 12
    physical inactivity, 12
    race, 11
    reducing, 12–13
    smoking, 11, 45–47
CVD, *see* Cerebrovascular
    disease
Cyanocobalamin, *see* Vitamin
    B$_{12}$
Cyclosporine–red yeast rice,
    interaction, 78

**D**

Daily value, 89
Dairy products
  calcium in, 37
  lowfat, 37
  vitamin D in, 37
Dementia, TIA-induced, 9
Depression, 69

Diabetes mellitus
  CAD risk, 12
  chromium therapy, 83–84
  exercise benefits, 43
  garlic, contraindications, 72
  niacin, contraindications, 64
  salt sensitivity, 126
  silent ischemia risk, 6
Diarrhea and vitamin C, 97
Diets, *see also* Foods
  angina association, 6
  Food Guide Pyramid, 26,
    35–37
  hypertension association, 126
  overview, 147
  typical American, 27
  vegetarian, 27
Dilantin–folic acid
  interactions, 112
Dioscorides, 66–67
Direct vasodilators,
  hypertension, 131–132
Disulfiram
  –niacin, interaction, 64
Diuretics, hypertension, 128–129
Dong Quai, cholesterol-
  lowering activities, 85
Dyslipidemias, *see also*
  Cholesterol
  description, 17

**E**

Edema, 8
EFAs, *see* Essential fatty acids
Eggs, limiting, 32
Electrocardiogram, 6
Endometrial cancer, ERT
  risks, 52–53

Endothelium, injury, 4
Epidemiologic studies,
  description, 56
ERT, *see* Estrogen-
  replacement therapy
Erythromycin–red yeast rice,
  interaction, 78
Essential fatty acids, *see* Fish
  oil; Flaxseed oil
Estrogen-replacement
  therapy, 52–53
Exercise
  angina treatment, 6
  benefits, 39–42
  CAD association, 12
  consistency, importance, 42
  daily activities as, 42
  frequency, 42–43
  hypertension benefits, 125
  overview, 147
  target heart rate, 44

**F**

Fats, *see also specific forms*
  AHA recommendations, 28,
    29–31
  blood, *see* Cholesterol
  content, label listing, 38–39
  –fiber association, 34–35
  nutrient absorption, 34
  trimming, tips, 40–41
  type diet, 27
  types, 29–31
  vegetarian diet, 27
Fatty streaks
  atherosclerosis marker, 4–5
  in children, 3
Fenofibrate, 51

Feverfew, cholesterol-lowering activities, 85

Fiber
  benefits, 33–34
  –fat association, 34–35
  types, 33–34

Fibrates
  description, 51
  –red yeast rice, interaction, 78

Fish oil
  blood pressure–lowering activity, 141, 153
  CAD, 81
  cholesterol lowering, 81–82
  overview, 149, 153

Flaxseed oil
  blood pressure–lowering activity, 142, 153
  CAD, 81
  overview, 153
  triglycerides, effectiveness, 82

Flushing, niacin side effect, 57, 61

Fluvastatin, 49

Folacin, *see* Folic acid

Folic acid
  CAD, 112–113
  description, 109–110
  dosage, 110–112
  food sources, 112
  fortification, 110
  homocysteine association, 104–109
  in multivitamins, 111
  overview, 150–151
  safety, 112

Food Guide Pyramid, 26, 35–37

Foods, *see also specific groups*
  antioxidants in, 101
  beta-carotene rich, 98–99, 100
  calcium rich, 137
  daily servings, 35–37
  folic acid
    fortification, 110
    rich, 112
  labels, 37–39
  magnesium rich, 137
  niacin rich, 60
  potassium rich, 137
  vitamin $B_6$ rich, 113
  vitamin $B_{12}$ rich, 114
  vitamin C rich, 95–96
  vitamin E rich, 93

Framingham Heart Study, 106
  CHF risks, 7–8
  heart attack mortality, 7
  high cholesterol risks, 17

Free radicals, *see also* Antioxidants
  benefits, 87
  damage, 87
  endothelium injury, 4
  fat production, 32

Fruits, serving recommendations, 35

## G

Gallstones, fibrate side effect, 51

Gamma-tocopherol, *see* Vitamin E

Garlic
  blood pressure–lowering activity, 70, 140–141, 153
  CAD, 66–73
  cholesterol and, 66–74

description, 67–68
dosage, 71–72
–ginkgo, interaction, 73
history, 66–67
mechanism, 71
overview, 148
safety, 72–73
studies, 68–70
–vitamin E, interaction, 73
Gemfibrozil, 51
Ginger, cholesterol-lowering
    activities, 85
Ginkgo
  cholesterol-lowering
      activities, 85
  –garlic, interaction, 73
  –vitamin E, interaction, 73
Glycosaminoglycans
      cholesterol-lowering
      activities, 82–83
Grape seed, cholesterol-
    lowering activities, 85
Green tea, cholesterol-
    lowering activities, 85
Gugulipid, cholesterol-
    lowering activity, 83

**H**

*H. pylori,* 3–4
Harvard Prospective Health
    Professional Follow-Up
    Study, 97
Hawthorn
  angina, 142, 153
  blood pressure–lowering
      activity, 142–143, 153
  CHF, 142
  cholesterol-lowering
      activities, 85

dosage, 143
overview, 153
safety, 144
studies, 142
HDL cholesterol
  description, 16
  levels, CAD risks, 22
  resin effects, 52
Heart attack
  beta-blockers,
      contraindications, 130
  description, 6
  CHF association, 7–8
  mortality rates, 6
  race, 7
  warning signs, 7
Heart disease, *see* Coronary
    artery disease
Heart palpitations, 143
Hemorrhagic stroke
  description, 8–9
  vitamin E risk, 93
Hepatitis, fibrate side
    effect, 51
Heredity, CAD risk, 11
High blood pressure, *see*
    Hypertension
High-density lipoproteins,
    *see also* HDL
    cholesterol
  description, 16
HMG-CoA reductase
    inhibitors, *see* Statins
Homocysteine
  B vitamin association,
      104–109, 150–151
  endothelium injury, 4
  levels, checking, 111
  risk factor, history, 103

Homocysteine (*continued*)
  studies
    B vitamin association,
      106–109
    risk factor, 104–105
Hormone-replacement
  therapy, 52
HRT, *see* Hormone-
  replacement therapy
Hydrogenation, 33
Hypercholesterolemia, *see*
  *also* Cholesterol
  associated risks, 17
  benefits of managing, 21–22
  CAD risk, 11
  conventional therapies
    diet, 26–39
      fats, 27–33, 147
      fiber, 33–35, 147
      Food Guide Pyramid, 26
      35–37
    exercise, 39–43, 147
    lipid-lowering drugs
      estrogen, 52–53
      fibrates, 51
      resins, 51–52
      statins, 49–51
    niacin, 55–65, 147–148
  incidence, 15, 25
  natural therapies
    bilberry, 85
    calcium, 84
    chromium, 83–84
    Dong Quai, 85
    EFAs, 81–82, 149
    feverfew, 85
    garlic, 66–74, 148
    ginger, 85

    ginkgo, 85
    glycosaminoglycans, 82–83
    grape seed, 85
    green tea, 85
    gugulipid, 83
    hawthorn, 85
    L-carnitine, 84
    lecithin, 84
    multivitamins, 85
    niacin, 55–65, 147–148
    pantethine, 83
    red yeast rice, 77–79,
      148–149
    sitostanol, 76, 148
    soy protein, 75–76, 148
    tocotrienols, 79–81, 149
    turmeric, 85
  NCEP guidelines, 20–21
  weight control, 43–44
Hyperglycemia, endothelium
  injury, 4
Hypertension
  angina association, 6
  CAD risk, 11–12
  causes, 118–119
  CHF association, 8
  chronic, 120
  classification, 121–123
  conventional therapies
    alcohol, moderation, 124
    diet, 125
    drugs
      ACE inhibitors, 129–130
      alpha-blockers, 130–131
      angiotensin II receptor-
      blockers, 130
      beta-blockers, 130
      calcium antagonists, 131

considerations, 132
direct vasodilators, 131–132
diuretics, 128–129
dose reduction, 127–128
side effects, 127
exercise, 41–42, 125
lifestyle modification
check list, 125
importance, 123
overview, 151
salt, limiting, 126
smoking cessation, 124
weight loss, 124–125
damage, 119–120
description, 8, 116–118
incidence, 115
monitoring, 115
mortality, 121
natural therapies
calcium, 136, 152
CoQ$_{10}$, 137–138, 152
EFAs, 81, 141–142, 153
garlic, 70, 140–141, 153
hawthorn, 142–143, 153
magnesium, 135–136, 152
potassium, 126–127, 135, 152
religious belief, 128
primary, description, 116–117
risk groups, 117
secondary, 116–117
description, 116–117
diagnosing, 134
stage I, definition, 117
"white coat," 118
Hypokalemia, 129
Hypotension, 129–130

**I**

Ibuprofen, for flushing reaction, 61
Immunosuppressive agents, 78
Insomnia, garlic side effect, 72
Insulin
chromium, effects, 83
exercise effects, 42
obesity effects, 43
Intermittent claudication, description, 2–3
Ischemia, silent, description, 6
Ischemic stroke, description, 8–9

**J**

JNC VI, 121, 123
Joint National Committee on Prevention, Detection, Evaluation, and Treatment of High Blood Pressure, 121, 123

**K**

Kidney
artery walls, 119
stones, vitamin C risks, 97

**L**

L-carnitine, cholesterol-lowering activity, 84
LDL cholesterol
AHA diet effects, 28–29
description, 16

LDL cholesterol (*continued*)
  drug therapy
    ERT, 52–53
    fibrates, 51
    resins, 51–52
    statins, 49–51
  drug therapy, based on, 21
  NCEP guidelines, 23
  plaque growth association,
    4–5
Lecithin, cholesterol-lowering
    activity, 84
Lescol, 49
Levodopa–vitamin B$_6$
    interaction, 113
Linolenic acid, blood
    pressure–lowering
    activity, 142
Lipid-lowering drugs
  benefits, 48–49
  NCEP guidelines, 23
  niacin and, 64
  types
    ERT, 52–53
    fibrates, 51
    resins, 51–52
    statins, 49–51
Lipitor, 49
Lipoproteins, *see* High-
    density lipoproteins;
    Low-density lipoproteins
Liver disease
  niacin, contraindications,
    61–64
  red yeast rice,
    contraindications, 78
Lopid, 51
Lovastatin, 49

Low-density lipoproteins, *see
    also* LDL cholesterol
  description, 16
Lung cancer
  beta-carotene risks, 98–100
  smoking risks, 46

# M

Magnesium
  blood pressuring–lowering
    effects, 135–136, 152
  daily value, 137
  food sources, 137
Margarine
  forms, 33
  manufacturing, 33
Meats
  lowfat, 41
  serving recommendations,
    35
Mevacor, 49
Minerals, *see specific types*
*Monascus purpureus, see* Red
    yeast rice
Monounsaturated fats,
    description, 31–32
Mortality, race, 7
MRFIT, *see* Multiple Risk
    Factor Intervention Trial
Mukul myrrh tree, *see*
    Gugulipid
Multiple Risk Factor Inter-
    vention Trial, 17–18
Multivitamins
  cholesterol-lowering
    activities, 85
  folic acid content, 111
  vitamin E content, 91–92

Myocardial infarction, *see* Heart attack

## N

National Cholesterol Education Program, guidelines, 20–21
Niacin
cholesterol and, 55–65, 147–148
description, 57
dosage, 59–60
flushing side effect, 57–61
flushless, 60
food sources, 60
overview, 147–148
–red yeast rice, interaction, 78
safety, 60–64
side effects, 57, 60–61
slow release, 61
statins *vs.*, 57
studies, 58–59
Niacinamide, 57
Nurses' Healthy Study, 107

## O

Obesity
CAD risk, 12
dangers, 43–44
hypertension risk, 124–125
Olive oil, benefits, 32
Omega-3 fatty acids, *see* Fish oil; Flaxseed oil
Organ transplants
garlic, contraindications, 72
red yeast rice contraindications, 78

Osteoporosis, 51
Oxidation, *see* Free radicals

## P

PAD, *see* Peripheral arterial disease
Palpitations, 143
Pantethine, cholesterol-lowering activity, 83
Parkinson's disease, *see* Levodopa–vitamin $B_6$, interaction
Peanut oil, benefits, 32
Pemphigus, garlic-induced, 72
Periodontitis, 4
Peripheral arterial disease, description, 2
Phenytoin–folic acid interactions, 112
Phosphatidylcholine, lecithin source, 84
Plaques, *see also* Atherosclerosis
build-up
acceleration, 3
process, 2
in children, 3
cholesterol role, 15
complicated, 5
dislodged, 5
Polyunsaturated fats
description, 31, 32–33
oxidation, 32
Pooling, blood, 8
Population studies, *see* Epidemiologic studies
Population study, description, 56

Potassium
  blood pressure–lowering
    effects, 135, 152
  daily value, 137
  food sources, 137
  high levels, effects, 30
  hypertension, 126–127
  low levels, effects, 129
Pravachol, 49
Pravastatin, 49
Prevention
  definitions, v
  types, v–vi
Prostaglandins, 61
Prozac, 69
Psyllium, 34
Pyridoxine, *see* Vitamin B<sub>6</sub>

## Q

Questran, 51

## R

Race
  CAD risk, 11
  heart attack mortality, 7
  hypertension, 117
Red wine, *see* Resveratrol
Red yeast rice
  cholesterol-lowering activity,
    77–79, 148–149
  –cyclosporine, interaction, 78
  description, 77
  dosage, 78
  –erythromycin, interaction,
    78
  –fibrates, interaction, 78
  –niacin, interaction, 78
  overview, 148–149

  safety, 78
  –statin, interaction, 78
  studies, 77–78
Religious belief, 128
Resins, *see* Bile acid
  sequestrants
Resveratrol, 101
Retina, artery walls, 119
Rice bran, *see* Tocotrienols
Risk factors
  aging, 10
  cholesterol levels, 11
  diabetes, 12
  gender, 11
  heredity, 11
  hypertension, 11–12
  reducing, 12–13
Roughage, *see* Fiber

## S

Salt sensitivity, hypertension
  and, 126
Saturated fats, description, 31
Scandinavian Simvastatin
  Survival Study, 50
Secondary prevention,
  definition, v
Silent ischemia, description, 6
Simvastatin, 49
Sitostanol
  cholesterol-lowering
    activity, 76
  margarine containing, 33
  overview, 148
Smoking
  angina association, 6
  beta-carotene, supplement,
    98–100

CAD risks, 11, 45–47
endothelium injury, 4
fish and, 81–82
Soy protein
cholesterol-lowering activity,
75–76
overview, 148
Statins
description, 49–51
–red yeast rice,
interaction, 78
Statistical significance, 59
Stroke
atherosclerosis association, 8
description, 8
incidence, 9
mortality, 9–10
types, 8–9
warning signs, 9

**T**

Target heart rate, 44
Teeth damage, vitamin C
risks, 97
Thrombi
formation, 5
inhibition, vitamin E, 91, 93
Tobacco smoking,
*see* Smoking
Tocopherol, *see* Vitamin E
Tocotrienol
cholesterol-lowering activity,
79–81, 149
dosage, 80
overview, 149
safety, 80–81
studies, 79–80
Tofu, *see* Soy protein

Trans-fatty acids, production,
33
Transplants
garlic, contraindication, 73
red yeast rice,
contraindication, 79
Triglycerides
description, 17
lowering
garlic, 69
pantethine, 83
Tryptophan, 57
Turmeric, cholesterol-
lowering activities, 85

**U**

Ubiquinone, *see*
Coenzyme $Q_{10}$
Uric acid levels, niacin
effects, 61

**V**

Vasodilators, direct,
hypertension, 132
Vegetables
lowfat, 41
serving recommendations, 35
Vegetarianism, 27
Very-low-density lipoprotein, 49
Vitamin A, *see also* Beta-
carotene
absorption, fat role, 34
production, 97
Vitamin $B_3$, *see* Niacin
Vitamin $B_6$
CAD, 105–109
description, 112–113
dosage, 113

Vitamin B$_6$ (*continued*)
  food sources, 113
  homocysteine association,
    104–109
  overview, 150–151
  safety, 113
Vitamin B$_{12}$
  CAD, 105–109
  description, 113
  dosage, 114
  food sources, 114
  homocysteine association,
    104–109
  overview, 150–151
Vitamin C
  CAD, 149–150
  description, 93
  dosage, 95–96
  food sources, 95–96
  overview, 150
  safety, 96–97
  studies, 95
  –vitamin E, benefits, 89–90
Vitamin D
  absorption, fat role, 34
  in dairy products, 37
Vitamin E
  absorption, fat role, 34
  alpha-tocopherol, 92, 95
  CAD, 89–92, 149–150
  deficiency, 88

  description, 88
  dosage, 90–91
  food sources, 93–94
  gamma-tocopherol, 95
  –garlic, interaction, 73
  –ginkgo, interaction, 73
  mechanism, 90–91
  natural, 92, 94–95
  overview, 149–150
  safety, 94–95
  studies, 88–91
  synthetic, 92, 94–95
  tocopherols, mixed, 95
  tocotrienols, inhibition, 80
  –vitamin C, benefits,
    89–90
Vitamin K absorption, 34
Vitamins content, label
    listing, 39

**W**

Weight loss, *see* Obesity
Wine, *see* Resveratrol
Women
  B vitamin therapy,
    107–109
  CAD risk, 11
  ERT, benefits, 52–53

**Z**

Zocor, 49

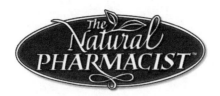

## About the Series Editors

**Richard Harkness, Pharm., FASCP,** an honors graduate of the Northeast Louisiana University School of Pharmacy, is a consultant pharmacist and a certified smoking cessation specialist. A nationally syndicated columnist, public speaker, and teacher, he is the author of *Drug Interactions Guide Book* (Prentice-Hall), *Drug Interactions Handbook* (Prentice-Hall), *OTC Handbook: What to Recommend & Why* (Medical Economics Co.), and *The Natural Pharmacist Guide to Reducing Cancer Risk* (Prima).

## About the Series Editors

**Steven Bratman, M.D.,** medical director of Prima Health, has many years of experience in the alternative medicine field. A graduate of the University of California at Davis, Medical School, he has also trained in herbology, nutrition, Chinese medicine, and other alternative therapies, and has worked closely with a wide variety of alternative practitioners. He is the author of *The Natural Pharmacist: Your Complete Guide to Herbs* (Prima), *The Natural Pharmacist: Your Complete Guide to Illnesses and Their Natural Remedies* (Prima), *The Alternative Medicine Ratings Guide* (Prima), and *The Alternative Medicine Sourcebook* (Lowell House).

**David J. Kroll, Ph.D.,** is a professor of pharmacology and toxicology at the University of Colorado School of Pharmacy and a consultant for pharmacists, physicians, and alternative practitioners on the indications and cautions for herbal medicine use. A graduate of both the University of Florida and the Philadelphia College of Pharmacy and Science, Dr. Kroll has lectured widely and has published articles in a number of medical journals, abstracts, and newsletters.